Cardiac CT Angiography Manual

Robert Pelberg and Wojciech Mazur

Cardiac CT Angiography Manual

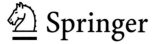 Springer

Robert Pelberg, MD, FACC
Wojciech Mazur, MD, FACC
The Ohio Heart and Vascular Center
Middletown, OH
USA

British Library Cataloguing in Publication Data

Pelberg, Robert
    Cardiac CT angiography manual
    1. Heart—Tomography   2. Angiocardiography
    I. Title   II. Wojciech, Mazur
    616.1′2′0757

    ISBN-13: 9781846286742

Library of Congress Control Number: 2006940056

ISBN-10: 1-84628-674-3   e-ISBN-10: 1-84628-675-1
ISBN-13: 978-1-84628-674-2   e-ISBN-13: 978-1-84628-675-9

Printed on acid-free paper

© Springer-Verlag London Limited 2007

9 8 7 6 5 4 3 2 1

Springer Science+Business Media
springer.com

Foreword

The *Cardiac CT Angiography Manual* is the first book of its kind; it is a handbook with concise and practical information related to the performance and interpretation of cardiac CT. I have known Dr. Pelberg since he entered this field, and I am quite honored to be able to provide this foreword. The editors are to be congratulated on presenting the most up-to-date, scientific, clinical, and particularly technical aspects of cardiac CT in a handbook format. The subject of this text is very timely given the current enthusiasm for cardiac CT and the large number of clinicians who are flocking to the field. The authors have compiled a list of important information, clinical pearls, and references. I know this will be another significant contribution to the field and will be seen as a "must have" in every lab performing cardiac CT today.

I have been blessed to be able to grow with the evolution of cardiac CT, and it is pleasing to see where we have arrived with 64 detector CT. This will be yet another significant contribution, making learning cardiac CT even easier than it has been to now.

Matthew Budoff, MD
Founding Board Member of the Society of Cardiovascular
Computed Tomography
President, Society of Atherosclerotic Imaging and Prevention
Harbor-UCLA, Torrance, CA

Preface

The *Cardiac CT Angiography Manual* was written for the purpose of making the exciting new field of cardiac computed tomography and calcium scoring simpler and more enjoyable to learn. It is intended to be a useful summary of the field of cardiac computed tomographic angiography (CTA) and calcium scoring that may aid in the training process. It is not meant to replace formal, hands-on training in this field. Difficult concepts are simplified, and figures are depicted for the purposes of clarity and understanding. The information was collected and compiled from peer-reviewed literature, lectures, and textbooks of cardiac CTA. In addition, we have tried to document the experiences and tips we have learned from the many visiting fellowships and courses we attended. Finally, we have also included information from our personal experience in performing this technique. We have attempted to be as complete as possible in documenting the sources of our information.

Cardiac CTA is a relatively new field that is constantly evolving and improving. New research and clinical experience are rapidly changing this technique. The authors believe the information in this book to be reliable and in accord with the standards accepted at the time that the document was written. However, in view of the possibility of human error or changes in the field, the authors do not warrant that the information contained herein is in every respect accurate or complete and they are not responsible for any errors or omissions, or for the results obtained from the use of such information. Readers are encouraged to confirm the information herein with other sources. For example, and in particular, readers are advised to check the product information sheet included in the package of each drug and contrast agent they plan to administer to be certain that information contained in this document is accurate and that changes have not been made in the recommended dose or in the contraindications for administration. In addition, readers are encouraged to be familiar with the concepts of radiation safety.

Robert Pelberg
Wojciech Mazur

Contents

Section I Calcium Scoring

1. Introduction to Calcium Scoring

Calcified coronary plaque represents approximately 20% of the total coronary artery plaque burden, and thus, the more coronary calcium, the more atherosclerotic burden is present. The other 80% of the coronary plaque is fibrous plaque or lipid-rich (soft) plaque. Therefore, coronary calcium is a measure of a patient's atherosclerotic burden. Calcium appears in the early stages of coronary artery disease and is a measure of atherosclerosis itself and does not simply represent a marker of disease like the traditional Framingham risk factors such as age, hypertension, family history, hyperlipidemia, and diabetes. One hypothesis is that calcium in the coronary arteries may mean that there was at least one incidence of a healed soft-plaque rupture with inflammation.

The calcium score (CaSc) helps to determine if the patient has atherosclerosis or not: Are they "in the game"? If coronary artery disease is present, the CaSc will provide information on the extent of disease. Is the atherosclerotic burden mild or severe (a lot or a little)? In addition, the CaSc will also determine the likelihood of a significant stenosis and the degree to which the atherosclerotic process is progressing. Is the disease worsening or has it been stabilized?

The CaSc scan is an easy technique, with low radiation. It is a noncontrast scan in which the power is turned down to a minimum to reduce radiation exposure. Unlike the contrasted computed tomographic angiography (CTA) scan, nonoverlapping, thicker slices are used, which further reduces radiation exposure. Finally, prospective triggering (discussed later) may be used, thereby lowering the radiation exposure even further.

The basic elements of the CaSc scan include blocking the field of view to include the heart, and sides of the lungs, allowing visualization of the heart and pericardium to permit the assessment of the cardiac chamber sizes, valve calcification, and coronary calcification. Electron beam CT (EBCT), which traditionally was used for calcium scoring, is now a dying breed for cardiac applications. Although EBCT has better temporal resolution at the present time (50 ms) because there are no moving parts (x-ray beams deflected by mirrors), the spatial resolution is not nearly as good as multidetector CT (MDCT) because the collimators are too thick. Thus, MDCT is now being used more frequently to obtain a CaSc. MDCT correlation with EBCT is still pending.

The Agatston score is the EBCT-based scale used to quantify coronary calcification and has plentiful data to support its usefulness. It is based on the density measurements of the calcium. The Agatston score is reproducible to ±15%–20%. The reason the Agatston score is accurate only to ±15%–20% is that the density of the calcium is assigned a weighting factor (density score) in a stepwise manner that is not linear or continuous. As illustrated in Figure 1.1, an insignificantly different Hounsfield unit score could yield a significantly

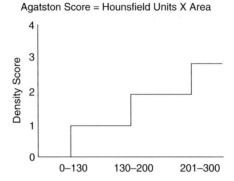

Agatston Score = Hounsfield Units X Area

Assume a calcium area of 5 pixels.
If the calcium measures 200 Hounsfield Units, the density score is 1.
If the calcium measures 201 Hounsfield Units, the density score is 2.
A density score of 1 X an area of 5 pixels yields an Agatston score of 5.
A density score of 2 X an area of 5 pixels yields an Agatston score of 10.
Therefore, an insignificant Hounsfield Unit difference yields a major Agatston score difference.

Figure 1.1. Stepwise relationship between Hounsfield units and the calcium density score as they relate to the determination of the Agatston score.

different density score. Because the Agatston score is a product of this density factor and the area of the calcium in the artery, a density score that is a factor higher will yield an Agatston score that is an order of magnitude different despite the fact that the Hounsfield unit scores for the calcium were very similar. For example, a Hounsfield unit score of 200 will result in a density factor of 1, whereas a score of 201 will yield a density score of 2. If the calcified area is 5 pixels, then the Hounsfield unit score of 200 will yield an Agatston score of 5 (product of a density score of 1 and a calcium area of 5 pixels). The Hounsfield unit score of 201 (not significantly different from a score of 200 as in the above example) will yield an Agatston score of 10 (product of a density score of 2 and a calcium area of 5 pixels) because the density factor was stepped up to 2 (Figure 1.1).

Other possible methods to measure coronary calcium include the calcium volume score and the calcium mass. The calcium volume score is more reproducible than the Agatston score, but partial volume effects may impair the accuracy of the volume score. Calcium mass, however, is accurate and demonstrates little variability but has a small database available to validate its use. Furthermore, the calcium mass is difficult to measure because it requires a phantom to be placed under the patient for calibrating purposes.

To be useful, the CaSc report must be clinically meaningful. In addition to positive or negative, the report must indicate a total score and the location of the calcium. For example, calcium in a critical location such as the left main coronary artery may have severe implications despite an overall low Agatston score. The report must also specify the likelihood of a tight lesion and provide an age percentile (age of the heart), which indicates the likelihood of cardiac events. The reader should also specify clinical recommendations. Does the patient need lifestyle modification, medications to reduce risk or further study (CTA, stress testing, nuclear imaging, or perhaps invasive coronary angiography)?

The calcium scan makes good economic and medical sense. Insurance will not pay for a cardiac CTA as a screen in asymptomatic patients at this time. Calcium scoring is a reasonable screen in this population because it is much cheaper and exposes the patient to significantly less radiation. Calcium scoring may be affordable to most patients. If the CaSc is positive, the resulting action (medications, nuclear stress testing, invasive angiography, or the CTA itself) will then likely be paid for by insurance. The CaSc can be scheduled on off times when the machine would otherwise not be in use. The test may be marketed to the community as an appropriate screening tool.

2. The Essentials of Calcium Scoring

There are five potential uses for coronary artery calcium scoring.

1.   To screen patients with moderate or intermediate Framingham risk. Positive calcium score (CaSc) scans will indicate incremental cardiac risk and may alter the therapeutic goals of treatment (low density lipoprotein, blood pressure, etc.). Because up to 50% of patients with myocardial infarction have no prodrome, early identification and treatment of high-risk patients is crucial (Figure 2.1) (D. Ropers, Department of Cardiology, University of Erlangen-Nurnberg, unpublished oral communication, April 6, 2006).

As a screening tool, CaSc is appropriate for asymptomatic patients with intermediate risk of coronary artery disease (10%–20% Framingham risk over 10 years) to help guide future management. The CaSc will either slide the patient upward to the high-risk group mandating treatment, or move them downward to the low-risk group, which would then preclude treatment. Intermediate-risk patients would include men 40–65 years of age with two or more risk factors and women 55–75 years of age with two or more risk factors. If an asymptomatic patient is young and possesses ≤1 risk factor, there is no advantage to a CaSc because their risk is already low. If an asymptomatic patient is high risk, they will be treated medically regardless of the CaSc. If symptoms are present, a diagnostic test is more appropriate than a screening test such as CaSc. These patients would be better suited for cardiac computed tomographic angiography (CTA), a stress test with or without nuclear imaging, or an invasive cardiac catheterization.

CaSc has also been determined to be an independent and incrementally more powerful risk factor for coronary events and mortality than the traditional Framingham risk indicators.[1] The PACC study[2] illustrated that in 2000 patients (mean age 43 years), coronary calcium was associated with an 11.8-fold increased risk for incident coronary heart disease. In young asymptomatic men, the presence of coronary artery calcification provided substantial, cost-effective, independent prognostic value in predicting incident coronary heart disease that was incremental to measured coronary risk factors (Figures 2.2 and 2.3).

All patients with any positive CaSc should be considered for medical therapy because a diagnosis of coronary artery disease has thus been made. If the CaSc is more than 100, patients should be considered for nuclear stress testing. These patients have a 2% per year likelihood of a coronary event and a 20% 10-year likelihood of a coronary event.[1,3] At a score of 100, there is a 20%–22% likelihood of a positive stress test;[1] that is, one in five will have silent ischemia. If the CaSc is less than 100 in an asymptomatic patient, the likelihood of a positive stress test is very low (2%–6% likelihood of a positive stress test),[1] and thus primary prevention is recommended without further testing. With scores between 100 and

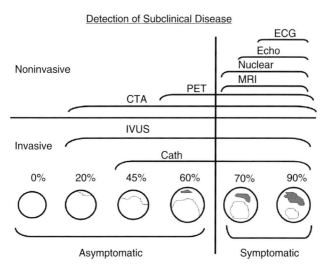

Figure 2.1. The various techniques available for the diagnosis of coronary atherosclerosis and their relationship to the extent of disease.

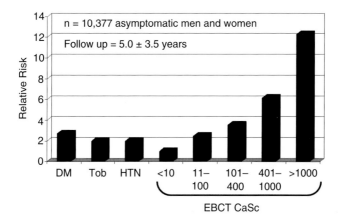

Figure 2.2. All-cause mortality in patients without known coronary artery disease. The graph demonstrates the impressive relative risk of all-cause mortality in relation to varying calcium scores and in relation to traditional cardiac risk factors. The relative risk of markedly increased calcium scores is exponentially greater than the relative risk of the more traditional cardiac risk factors. EBCT, electron beam computed tomography; DM, diabetes melitus; Tob, tobacco; HTN, hypertension. (Shaw et al.[4])

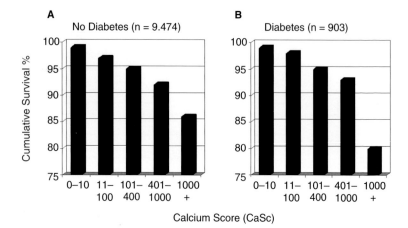

Figure 2.3. The relationship between 5 year percent cumulative survival and CaSc in both nondiabetics (**A**) and diabetics (**B**). The survival rate plummets in patients with extensive calcium. Conversely, those patients with very low CaSc (diabetic or nondiabetic) have a very good survival rate. (**A**, Shaw et al.[4]; **B**, Budoff, unpublished written communication, May 1, 2006.)

400, there is a gradual increase in the likelihood of a positive stress test. If the CaSc is 0, then the 10-year cardiovascular event rate is just 1%.[1] Because the risk of a statin is greater than 1% per year, if the CaSc is 0, a statin may not be required (Figure 2.4).

A CaSc of more than 400 would justify a nuclear stress test to determine the functional significance of the coronary artery disease (ischemic burden). Some say that patients with a CaSc more than 400 should be considered for invasive cardiac catheterization (Callister, The Tennessee Heart and Vascular Institute, unpublished oral communication, Novem-

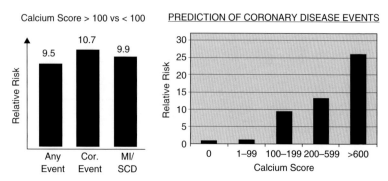

Figure 2.4. Two gr aphs from the St. Francis Heart Study depicting the relative risk of a coronary event in relation to varying calcium scores. As the calcium score increases, the risk of a cardiac event increases. Cor, coronary; MI/SCD, myocardial infarction/sudden cardiac death.

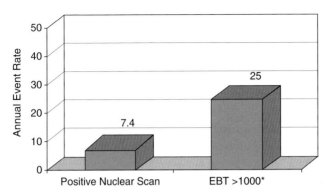

Figure 2.5. Prognostic significance of high calcium scores in asymptomatic persons.[10] The graph demonstrates the prognostic significance of a calcium score above 1000 related to a positive nuclear scan, indicating the power of a markedly increased CaSc. Calcium scoring may even be more predictive than a positive nuclear scan. EBT, electron beam tomography.

ber 4, 2005). A score of 400 or more represents a 45% likelihood of a positive stress test and the likelihood levels off at higher scores (Callister, The Tennessee Heart and Vascular Institute, unpublished oral communication, November 4, 2005). Because it is a coin flip (50 : 50) as to whether one has a tight lesion with a CaSc, some believe it is reasonable to proceed to catheterization (Callister, The Tennessee Heart and Vascular Institute, unpublished oral communication, November 4, 2005). This approach would be very aggressive. Most others believe a score of 1000 or more would be required to justify invasive cardiac catheterization. A CaSc of greater than 1000 may be more predictive of a negative outcome than a positive nuclear scan (Figure 2.5).[10] There is no consensus that an invasive angiogram is ever indicated on the basis of a CaSc alone without an abnormal functional study. Table 2.1 and Figure 2.6 depict possible clinical algorithms based on the CaSc.

Diabetics have a vastly greater cardiac risk at any given CaSc. However, a diabetic with a CaSc of 0 falls into a much lower risk group than the

Table 2.1. Possible algorithm #1*: a possible algorithm for how to clinically react to various calcium scores

CaSc	Action
0	Consider repeat screening
1–100	Medical management
101–399	Meds plus nuclear stress
≥400	Meds plus nuclear stress versus catheterization

* Callister, The Tennessee Heart and Vascular Institute, unpublished written communication, November 4, 2005.

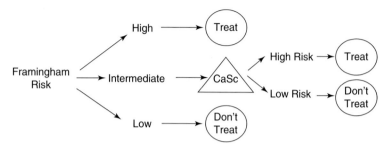

Figure 2.6. Possible algorithm #2 (Budoff, UCLA Medical Center, Los Angeles, CA, unpublished oral communication, May 1, 2006): an alternative clinical algorithm regarding calcium scoring, which takes into account traditional Framingham risk.

usual diabetic. These findings are illustrated in Figure 2.3B. At the present time, however, the American College of Cardiology recommends that all diabetics be treated as if they already have coronary artery disease. It should also be noted that African American patients have half as much calcium as Caucasians, yet they have more cardiac events.

2.   To identify patients who do not need further cardiac evaluation (scores of 0). In addition to screening, CaSc is very useful in eliminating patients from further testing and treatment. The negative predictive value of CaSc is very powerful. Zero scores have a 95%–99% negative predictive power.[5-7] Knez et al.[8] studied 2115 persons with CaSc before invasive angiography and determined that calcium was present in more than 99% of patients with obstructive coronary artery disease. No calcium was found in eight patients who had significant luminal stenoses (7 of 872 men or 0.7% and 1 of 383 women or 0.02%). Seven of the eight patients with missed obstructive disease and scores of 0 were <45 years old. This study yielded a negative predictive value of >99%, indicating that CaSc may potentially be used as a filter before invasive angiography to help avoid negative angiograms. In younger patients (≤40 years), this negative predictive power breaks down because younger patients have less time to calcify and tend to have more soft plaque and clot-laden, tight stenoses.

In addition, the Mayo Clinic Chest Pain Unit[9] used electron beam computed tomography to screen 100 patients ≥40 years of age who presented to the emergency room with chest pain. Fifty percent were women and 98% were Caucasian. All future events occurred in patients with coronary calcium. Based on other independent testing, of those with diagnosed coronary disease, 14 had a CaSc of >0 and zero had a CaSc of 0. Of those not found to have coronary disease, 32 had a positive CaSc and 54 had a CaSc of 0, yielding a sensitivity of 100% for the CaSc in identifying those with coronary artery disease, and a specificity of 63%. However, the negative predictive value for significant coronary artery disease was 100%. All events occurred in patients with calcium and no events occurred in patients without calcium.

It is, however, important to understand the limitations of the CaSc. If the CaSc is 0 and the patient is ≥40 years of age, there is only a 1 in 2000 chance of finding a high-grade lesion on invasive angiography. This is not to say that there is no disease, however. The CaSc is, therefore, very good at ruling out significant obstructive coronary artery disease. After the age of 65 years, the CaSc may become less predictive because most patients have coronary calcium. Therefore, the difference in the calcium scores of patients with and without coronary events is not as great as in those who are between 40 to 65 years of age (Budoff, UCLA Medical Center, Los Angeles, CA, unpublished oral communication, May 1, 2006). In patients ≤45 years of age, the negative predictive value of the CaSc breaks down as noted by Knez et al.[8]

CaSc may also be used to evaluate a cardiomyopathy of unknown etiology. The sensitivity of coronary calcium in identifying an ischemic cardiomyopathy is 99%,[11] where a positive CaSc suggests an ischemic etiology. Studies[11–13] suggest that the CaSc is a stronger predictor of an ischemic etiology for cardio-myopathy than echocardiography, stress testing, and stress nuclear at distinguishing ischemic from nonischemic cardiomyopathy,[11–13] and thus may prevent the need for further testing for this indication.

3. To assess disease progression with serial imaging. Calcium scoring may also be used longitudinally to serially image patients in evaluating the rate of progression of disease. It is reasonable to repeat scanning on negative scores (CaSc = 0) every 3 years for diabetics and every 5 years for all others. If the score is 0, the cardiovascular risk over the next several years will be very low. A score of 0 does not, however, guarantee absence of disease, but rather that the patient has a very low disease burden, if any disease at all, and that the chance for a tight stenosis is very low (but not 0). The CTA itself will diagnose disease (soft plaque) with greater sensitivity than the CaSc.

If the CaSc is positive, serial screening may indicate a progression of atherosclerosis that portends a markedly worsened prognosis. In Figure 2.7, Raggi et al.[14] demonstrated a markedly worsened prognosis if an individual CaSc changed by more than 15% in 1 year. All patients in this study were on statins. Therefore, calcium scoring may help to assess the effectiveness of statins (or other medical therapy).

The St. Francis Heart Study,[1] the largest study reported to date in this arena, demonstrated that only age ($P = .03$), male gender ($P = .04$), low density lipoprotein cholesterol ($P = .01$), high density lipoprotein cholesterol ($P = .04$), and a 2-year change in CaSc ($P = .0001$) were significantly associated with subsequent cardiac events.

A proposed formula to predict stabilization of CaSc is [(square root of initial CaSc) + time between score in years (i.e., 1.5) = acceptable rate of progression] (Callister, The Tennessee Heart and Vascular Institute, unpublished oral communication, November 4, 2005). If the repeat score is higher than this predicted score, then the atherosclerotic disease

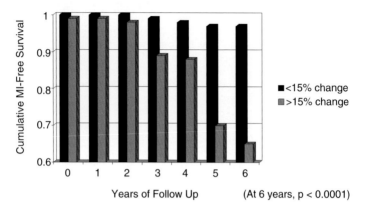

Figure 2.7. Time to acute myocardial infarction (MI) versus yearly CaSc change.[14] The graph depicts the importance of a change in calcium score over time. If the CaSc changes by more than 15% in a given year, the cumulative survival time free of MI markedly decreases.

process is not under control and the subsequent event rate is high (Callister, The Tennessee Heart and Vascular Institute, unpublished oral communication, November 4, 2005).

An emerging concept is that the vascular age or the "age of your heart" is of greater prognostic importance than the chronological age. CaSc tables have been developed to help assess the age of a patient's heart. These tables display the "age of the heart" in relation to the chronological age. For example, a heart may be "10 years older than it should be." This is a poor man's way of determining the rate of progression of disease. The CaSc may answer the question "Is this disease progressing quickly?" indicating a higher incidence of events than in those where the disease progression has stabilized. A score that places a patient into the 50th percentile means that the score is similar to 50% of patients of that age. If the CaSc is at the 90th percentile, the risk is higher because the disease is progressing faster since only 10% of patients have a higher CaSc. This is irrespective of total score. A fast progression of disease is a negative predictor, independent of total calcium burden, which is also a negative predictor (Tables 2.2–2.5).

Diagrams have also been developed to assess cardiovascular risk based on the vascular age (Figure 2.8) (Callister, The Tennessee Heart and Vascular Institute, unpublished written communication, November 4, 2005).
4.   To improve medical compliance. Patients are often not compliant with appropriate dietary practices, exercise regimes, smoking cessation advice, and medicine prescriptions. By demonstrating calcium in the coronary arteries, patients and physicians may be convinced to be more compliant with lifestyle modification and medical therapy for atherosclerosis. Kalia et al.[15] demonstrated that the higher the CaSc, the more likely the patient was to remain on statin therapy (Figure 2.9). It is not known

Table 2.2. Male CaSc age adjusted percentiles

Age (y)	Percentiles		
	50%	75%	90%
30–34	0	0	6
35–39	0	0	16
40–44	0	10	58
45–49	2	37	162
50–54	13	86	279
55–59	35	176	478
60–64	98	409	726
65–70	140	493	1095

Table 2.3. Female CaSc age adjusted percentiles

Age (y)	Percentiles		
	50%	75%	90%
30–34	0	0	0
35–39	0	0	2
40–44	0	0	8
45–49	0	0	22
50–54	0	6	55
55–59	0	29	132
60–64	3	59	261
65–70	14	103	338

Table 2.4. Female CaSc age adjusted percentiles

CaSc	Age (y)									
	35	40	45	50	55	60	65	70	75	80
0	10	10	10	10	10	10	10	10	10	10
1	80	75	70	60	50	40	30	30	30	30
3	80	80	75	60	60	40	40	30	30	30
5	90	80	75	70	60	50	40	30	30	30
7	90	80	80	70	70	50	50	40	30	30
12	90	80	80	75	70	60	50	40	30	30
15	95	90	80	75	75	60	50	40	40	30
25	95	90	80	80	80	60	60	50	40	30
50	95	90	90	80	80	70	60	50	50	30
75	95	95	90	80	80	75	70	60	50	40
100	95	95	90	90	80	80	75	60	60	40
125	95	95	95	90	80	80	75	60	60	50
150	95	95	95	90	90	80	80	70	60	50
200	95	95	95	90	90	80	80	75	70	60
300	95	95	95	95	95	90	80	80	75	70
400	95	95	95	95	95	90	90	80	80	75
500	95	95	95	95	95	95	90	90	80	75

(Continued)

Table 2.4. *Continued*

CaSc	Age (y)									
	35	40	45	50	55	60	65	70	75	80
600	95	95	95	95	95	95	95	90	80	80
700	95	95	95	95	95	95	95	90	90	80
800	95	95	95	95	95	95	95	90	90	80
900	95	95	95	95	95	95	95	95	90	90
1000	95	95	95	95	95	95	95	95	90	90
1200	95	95	95	95	95	95	95	95	95	90
1500	95	95	95	95	95	95	95	95	95	90
1800	95	95	95	95	95	95	95	95	95	95

Note: Data are in percentages.

Table 2.5. Male CaSc age adjusted percentiles

CaSc	Age (y)									
	35	40	45	50	55	60	65	70	75	80
0	10	10	10	10	10	10	10	10	10	10
1	70	50	40	30	20	20	20	20	20	20
3	75	60	50	40	30	20	20	20	20	20
5	75	70	60	40	30	20	20	20	20	20
7	80	75	60	50	40	30	20	20	20	20
12	80	75	70	50	40	30	30	20	20	20
15	90	80	75	60	50	30	30	20	20	20
25	95	80	75	60	50	40	30	30	20	20
50	95	90	80	70	60	50	40	30	30	20
75	95	90	80	75	60	50	50	40	30	30
100	95	95	90	80	70	60	50	40	40	30
150	95	95	90	80	75	60	60	50	50	30
200	95	95	95	90	80	70	60	50	50	40
300	95	95	95	90	80	75	70	60	50	40
400	95	95	95	95	90	80	75	70	60	50
500	95	95	95	95	90	80	80	75	70	60
600	95	95	95	95	95	80	80	75	70	60
700	95	95	95	95	95	90	80	80	75	70
800	95	95	95	95	95	90	90	80	75	70
900	95	95	95	95	95	95	90	80	80	75
1000	95	95	95	95	95	95	90	80	80	75
1200	95	95	95	95	95	95	95	90	80	75
1500	95	95	95	95	95	95	95	90	90	80
1800	95	95	95	95	95	95	95	95	90	90
2000	95	95	95	95	95	95	95	95	95	90
2200	95	95	95	95	95	95	95	95	95	95

Note: Data are in percentages.

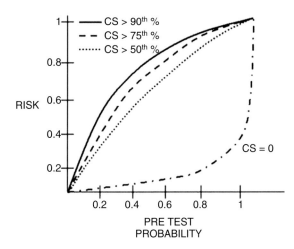

Figure 2.8. Risk lift (Callister, The Tennessee Heart and Vascular Institute, unpublished written communication, November 4, 2005). The relationship between pretest probability of coronary artery disease and CaSc percentile as it affects clinical risk. The risk of coronary artery disease is markedly higher (at any pretest probability) the greater the CaSc percentile. CS, calcium score.

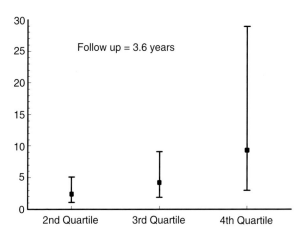

Figure 2.9. Odds ratio of maintaining statin Rx with various levels of baseline calcium[15] (Budoff, UCLA Medical Center, Los Angeles, CA, unpublished oral communication, May 1, 2006). This graph indicates that as the calcium score quartile increases, the likelihood of medical compliance increases.

whether this finding represents better patient compliance with the physician recommendations or stricter physician adherence to guidelines based on the knowledge that coronary artery disease is already present.

5.   To serve as an adjunct to noninvasive coronary computed tomographic angiography (CTA). A CaSc of 0 has a 96%–99% negative predictive power of future cardiac events. Patients with extremely high scores, however, often have nondiagnostic CTA images because the calcium may obscure visualization of the coronary lumens. Therefore, the CaSc may be used to screen for those that should and should not move on to CTA. In general, a CaSc of >1000 should not have a CTA performed because of the high likelihood of an unreadable scan. This is not always the case, however, because it is not necessarily the amount of calcium that will hinder the diagnostic value of the CTA, but rather the location of the calcium (diffuse or focal calcification). Diffuse calcification will render a CTA less likely to be diagnostic. In addition, the location of the calcium may also be of prognostic value despite a low score (left main calcium).

In addition, the noncontrasted scan may help to plan the field of view for the CTA. It may also allow a test run for breath holding and to check for heart rate variability during the breath hold before the contrasted scan.

Finally, calcification in other structures of the chest may be detected as well. Other important areas of calcification to observe include aortic calcification, aortic valve calcification, mitral annular calcification, myocardial calcification, and pericardial calcification. There are emerging data that aortic valve calcification and scoring may aid in determining the severity of aortic stenosis.[16]

In summary, CaSc for risk stratification seems to be a powerful tool in the clinically selected intermediate-risk population. Soft plaque will add to the prognostic information. Zero scores in patients over the age of 40 likely do not need any further cardiac evaluations. The CaSc can track the progression of disease and stimulate compliance. Because all the prognostic data have been published in 2005 or later, there is a lag between the data and insurance companies' willingness to pay for this screening test.

Section II Cardiac CTA

3. Indications for Cardiac CTA

Cardiac catheterization remains the gold standard for diagnosing coronary artery disease. Invasive angiography has excellent spatial and temporal resolution, and coronary intervention may often be done at the same sitting. However, cardiac catheterization is invasive and fails to visualize the vessel wall. Because it is a representation of the lumen only, cardiac catheterization does not visualize soft plaque. Invasive angiography also underestimates atherosclerotic burden, especially in a positively remodeled vessel. Intravascular ultrasound is cumbersome and has its own limitations, difficulties, and costs.

Computed tomographic coronary angiography is ideal for screening moderate-risk patients for atherosclerotic coronary artery disease, for determining atherosclerotic disease burden, for evaluating patients suspected to have coronary anomalies, and for an alternative to invasive angiography in stable patients as a means of determining atherosclerotic disease burden. In addition, computed tomographic coronary angiography may be used to plan a strategy for revascularization.

Potential indications for computed tomography angiography (CTA) would include many categories and these indications continue to evolve. Listed below is a suggested list of potential indications for cardiac CTA.

1. After stress test imaging where the stress test is equivocal, positive but without high-risk characteristics, or negative but significant symptoms persist. In this case, CTA would be used to absolutely rule out significant coronary artery disease or to discover another significant cause of symptoms other than coronary artery disease.
2. In the evaluation of chest pain when the electrocardiogram is uninterpretable and the patient cannot exercise.
3. In the evaluation of low-risk patients with chest pain in the emergency room setting.
4. To assess risk in the general population with moderate or high Framingham risk.
5. To further assess high calcium scores of greater than 400. It is controversial whether a CTA should be performed if the calcium score is more than 1000.
6. In the assessment of patients scheduled to undergo noncoronary cardiac surgery such as valve surgery.
7. In the preoperative risk assessment for noncardiac surgery if intermediate or high-risk surgery is planned.
8. To evaluate a patient after angioplasty or stenting. There are limited data in this area, but CTA may be useful in selected patients if the stent diameter is greater than 3.5 mm.
9. To evaluate patients with increased risk of complications from coronary angiography (increased risk of stroke, poor vascular access, or are taking coumadin, etc.).

10. To evaluate patients with suspected coronary anomalies. CTA may be helpful to define whether an anomalous coronary artery takes an intramural or an extramural course (see explanation below) or whether the anomalous artery travels between the great vessels or around the great vessels.

11. After incomplete catheterization [i.e., left internal mammary artery (LIMA) not visualized] and to help with percutaneous intervention. The CTA may help catheter selection to allow appropriate backup support by allowing accurate characterization and sizing of the aortic root. The majority of the anatomic attributes of the lesion can be characterized by CTA as well to gauge the probability of success and the risk of the procedure. Computerized gantry coordinates can aid in optimizing catheterization views to save dye. This may also reduce radiation exposure for the patient and operator. In addition, because CTA is not artery selective, collateral flow may allow better imaging of the distal vessels.

12. In patients undergoing electrophysiology procedures to define cardiac vein anatomy before biventricular pacing (i.e., coronary vein mapping). To assess the heart before atrial fibrillation ablation in selected patients in order to define pulmonary venous anatomy, measure the left atrial size, and rule out left atrial appendage thrombus. Pulmonary veins and the left atrium proper can easily be visualized in the presence of atrial fibrillation but sinus rhythm may be necessary to visualize the left atrial appendage. CTA may also be useful in the assessment of the post–atrial fibrillation ablation follow-up to check for pulmonary vein stenosis.

13. In the screening evaluation of coronaries after heart transplantation.

14. To determine bypass graft patency in selected patients.

15. To define abnormal echocardiographic findings such as pericardial cysts, partial absence of the left pericardium, coronary fistulas and shunt anatomy, cardiac masses and tumors, thrombus, cinefluoroscopy of mechanical heart valves for thrombosis and pannus and decreased mobility, endocarditis (vegetations and abscesses), and left ventricular apical thrombus determination (clot is +50 Hounsfield units).

16. To plan a redo coronary bypass surgery. CTA may help identify the location of the LIMA beneath the sternum. Be sure the scan field is adequate to include the LIMA. CTA may also help to plan coronary angiogram and aortic cross-clamping approach depending on the extent or location of aortic calcified atheroma.

17. May help plan the best route for cardiac catheterization in difficult cases to identify the ostia of the coronary arteries.

18. In aortic dissection, CTA might help assess the path for angiography, by identifying the true and false lumen and from which lumen the coronaries arise.

19. To assess the etiology of cardiomyopathy (ischemic versus nonischemic).

20. In congenital heart disease. CTA is an excellent test for morphology and structure.
21. To evaluate cardiac function in patients with poor echocardiographic windows.
22. To evaluate motion of a mechanical valve if malfunction is suspected. This test is much better than fluoroscopy for this purpose.
23. In the evaluation of native or prosthetic valves in general if transesophageal echocardiography or transthoracic echocardiography is not diagnostic. Keep in mind that computed tomography does not at this time replace echocardiography for assessment of valvular heart disease. To date, CTA has only been validated to be useful in aortic valve planimetry for aortic stenosis.
24. In the evaluation for aortic dissection.
25. In the evaluation for pulmonary embolism.

Recently, the American College of Cardiology Foundation Quality Strategic Directions Committee Appropriateness Criteria Working Group, the American College of Radiology, the Society of Cardiovascular Computed Tomography, The Society for Cardiovascular Magnetic Resonance, the American Society of Nuclear Cardiology, the North American Society for Cardiac Imaging, the Society for Cardiovascular Angiography and Interventions, and the Society of Interventional Radiology published a joint review on the appropriateness of cardiac CTA.[17] This report "critically and systematically"[17] reviewed the appropriateness of cardiac CTA and after assessing the risks and benefits of cardiac CTA for several clinical indications scored these indications on a scale of 1 to 9 where a score of 7 to 9 suggests a generally acceptable indication, a score of 4 to 6 represents indications whose benefit and appropriateness are at this time uncertain, and a score of 1 to 3 generally implies an inappropriate indication.

Tables 3.1–3.3 list the appropriateness criteria as published by the cardiac computed tomography and cardiac magnetic resonance writing groups.[17] The database on cardiac CTA at this time is in development and is not currently robust enough to support categorical recommendations in the form of formal guidelines. The appropriateness criteria are not guidelines, but rather an intermediate position before the publication of official guidelines which certainly will follow as the database on cardiac CTA becomes more complete.

Table 3.1. Appropriate indications (score of 7–9)[17]

Indication	Appropriateness criteria score
Detection of CAD: symptomatic—evaluation of chest pain syndrome	
1. • Intermediate pretest probability of CAD	A (7)
• Uninterpretable ECG or unable to exercise	
Detection of CAD: symptomatic—evaluation of intracardiac structures	
2. • Evaluation of suspected coronary anomalies	A (9)
Detection of CAD: symptomatic—acute chest pain	
3. • Intermediate pretest probability of CAD	A (7)
• No ECG changes and serial enzymes negative	
Detection of CAD with prior test results—evaluation of chest pain syndrome	
4. • Uninterpretable or equivocal stress test (exercise, perfusion, or stress echo)	A (8)
Structure and function—morphology	
5. • Assessment of complex congenital heart disease including anomalies of coronary circulation, great vessels, and cardiac chambers and valves	A (7)
6. • Evaluation of coronary arteries in patients with new onset heart failure to assess etiology	A (7)
Structure and function—evaluation of intra- and extracardiac structures	
7. • Evaluation of suspected cardiac mass (tumor or thrombus)	A (8)
• Patients with technically limited images from echo, MRI, or TEE	
8. • Evaluation of pericardial conditions (pericardial mass, constrictive pericarditis, or complications of cardiac surgery	A (8)
• Patients with technically limited images from echo, MRI, or TEE	
9. • Evaluation of pulmonary vein anatomy before invasive radiofrequency ablation for atrial fibrillation	A (8)
10. • Noninvasive coronary vein mapping before placement of biventricular pacemaker	A (8)
11. • Noninvasive coronary arterial mapping, including internal mammary artery before repeat cardiac revascularization	A (8)
Structure and function—evaluation of aortic and pulmonary disease	
12. • Evaluation of suspected aortic dissection or aneurysm	A (9)
13. • Evaluation of suspected pulmonary embolism	A (9)

A, appropriate; ECG, electrocardiogram; MRI, magnetic resonance imaging; TEE, transesophageal echocardiography.

Table 3.2. Uncertain indications (score of 4–6)[17]

Indication	Appropriateness criteria score
Detection of CAD: symptomatic—evaluation of chest pain syndrome	
1. • Intermediate pretest probability of CAD • ECG interpretable *and* able to exercise	U (5)
Detection of CAD: symptomatic—acute chest pain	
2. • Low pretest probability of CAD • No ECG changes and serial enzymes negative	U (5)
3. • High pretest probability of CAD • No ECG changes and serial enzymes negative	U (6)
4. • "Triple rule out"—exclude obstructive CAD, aortic dissection, and pulmonary embolism • Intermediate pretest probability for one of the above • ECG—no ST segment elevation and initial enzymes negative	U (4)
Detection of CAD: asymptomatic (without chest pain syndrome)	
5. • High CHD Framingham risk	U (4)
Risk assessment: general population—asymptomatic (calcium scoring)	
6. • Moderate CHD Framingham risk 7. • High CHD Framingham risk	U (5)
Risk assessment: preoperative evaluation for noncardiac surgery— intermediate- or high-risk surgery	
8. • Intermediate perioperative risk	U (4)
Detection of CAD: postrevascularization (PCI or CABG)— evaluation of chest pain syndrome	
9. • Evaluation of bypass grafts and coronary anatomy	U (6)
10. • History of percutaneous revascularization with stents	U (5)
Structure and function—evaluation of ventricular and valvular function	
11. • Evaluation of LV function after myocardial infarction *or* in heart failure patients • Patients with technically limited images from echo	U (5)
12. • Characterization of native and prosthetic cardiac valves • Patients with technically limited images from echo, MRI, or TEE	U(5)

ECG, electrocardiogram; CHD, coronary heart disease; PCI, percutaneous coronary intervention; CABG, coronary artery bypass graft; LV, left ventricular; MRI, magnetic resonance imaging; TEE, transesophageal echocardiography; U, uncertain.

Table 3.3. Inappropriate indications (score of 1–3)[17]

Indication	Appropriateness criteria score
Detection of CAD: symptomatic—evaluation of chest pain syndrome	
1. • High pretest probability of CAD	I (2)
Detection of CAD: symptomatic—acute chest pain	
2. • High pretest probability of CAD	I (1)
• ECG—ST segment elevation and/or positive cardiac enzymes	
Detection of CAD: asymptomatic (without chest pain syndrome)	
3. • Low CHD Framingham risk	I (1)
4. • Moderate CHD Framingham risk	I (2)
Risk assessment general population—asymptomatic (calcium scoring)	
5. • Low CHD Framingham risk	I (1)
Detection of CAD with prior test results—evaluation of chest pain syndrome	
6. • Evidence of moderate to severe ischemia on stress test (exercise, perfusion, or stress echo)	I (2)
Risk assessment with prior test results—asymptomatic (calcium scoring)	
7. • Prior calcium score within previous 5 years	I (1)
Risk assessment with prior test results—asymptomatic	
8. • High CHD Framingham risk	I (2)
• Within 2 years prior cardiac CT angiogram or invasive angiogram without significant obstructive disease	
9. • High CHD Framingham risk	I (3)
• Prior calcium score ≥400	
Risk assessment: preoperative evaluation for noncardiac surgery— low-risk surgery	
10. • Intermediate perioperative risk	I (1)
Detection of CAD: postrevascularization (PCI or CABG)—asymptomatic	
11. • Evaluation of bypass grafts and coronary anatomy	I (2)
• Less than 5 years after CABG	
12. • Evaluation of bypass grafts and coronary anatomy	I (3)
• ≥5 years after CABG	
13. • Evaluation for in-stent restenosis and coronary anatomy after PCI	I (2)
Structure and function: evaluation of ventricular and valvular function	
14. • Evaluation of LV function after myocardial infarction *or* in heart failure patients	I (3)

CHD, coronary heart disease; PCI, percutaneous coronary intervention; CABG, coronary artery bypass graft; I, inappropriate; LV, left ventricular.

4. General Overview of Cardiac CTA

Basic Requirements for Successful Cardiac CTA

The following is a general discussion on the requirements of cardiac computed tomographic angiography (CTA). Each of the elements in this general discussion will be described in more detail. Cardiac CTA requires high temporal resolution (time required to acquire one image) to minimize motion artifacts caused by cardiac motion and breathing. This requires a fast gantry rotation with multiple detectors. Because the coronaries are seen best when there is the least motion, the diastolic phase is most optimal for imaging and thus the temporal resolution must be less than the length of the diastolic phase (the goal is to try to freeze the heart in the diastolic phase). Currently, the fastest gantry rotation speed is 330 ms. The G force produced by this gantry rotation speed is approximately 28 Gs. A gantry rotation speed of <200 ms (required to provide a temporal resolution of 100 ms) would generate 75 Gs and is beyond today's technological limits (Figure 4.1) because there is no current material capable of containing an X-ray source and detector array moving at this speed.

Only a half-gantry rotation is needed to reconstruct the entire cardiac image and as such the effective temporal resolution for single-slice reconstruction (one slice reconstructed from half-gantry rotation) is 165 ms, which can be further reduced to 82.5 ms with multisegmental reconstruction (discussed below), albeit at the cost of potential misregistration artifacts. In dual-source CT, only a quarter-gantry rotation is necessary for cardiac imaging thus resulting in a temporal resolution of 82.5 ms without the need for multisegmental reconstruction and 60 ms if multisegmental reconstruction techniques are used.

High spatial resolution is also necessary to allow imaging of the coronary arteries, which are small, tortuous three-dimensional structures. Imaging the coronary arteries requires very thin collimation and the smallest focal point and detector size, with the shortest distance between detectors. In addition, isotropic voxels (three-dimensional pixels) of less than 1 mm are necessary. Isotropic voxels are voxels whose dimensions in the x-, y-axis (in-plane) and the z-axis (through-plane) are the same. Voxels with identical dimensions in all three planes (isotropic) allow for similar spatial resolution in all planes and thus permit analysis of the heart in all planes without image distortion or loss of integrity. The 64 detectors (isotropic) allow an x-, y-axis spatial resolution of near 0.4 mm. The z-axis spatial resolution or slice thickness is almost 0.6 mm.

Also required for successful cardiac CTA imaging is fast contiguous coverage of the heart to allow imaging of the entire heart in one breath hold. This requires the multislice helical CT technique (rotating gantry). Each slice of the

ROTATION SPEEDS

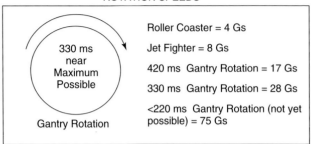

Figure 4.1. The force necessary to rotate the gantry at speeds required to yield clinically useful temporal resolution compared with more mundane examples.

heart is collected in one heartbeat (or two to four beats if various multisegmented reconstruction techniques are used). Generally, there is a 30%–50% overlap between each slice.

Finally, the scan must be synchronized or triggered to the heartbeat to allow gating so that the heart can be imaged in multiple slices across multiple heartbeats in the same phase. Each slice of the heart in the *z*-axis is then reconstructed at the same cardiac phase to, in essence, freeze the heart.

Accuracy of Cardiac CTA

Table 4.1 illustrates the sensitivity and specificity of scanners with various detector numbers. Although the sensitivity and specificity of the 16- versus the 64-slice scanners are similar, the percentage of segments that cannot be evaluated are reduced significantly with the 64-slice scanner.

Table 4.1. Sensitivity and specificity of cardiac CTA in relation to the number of detector rows*

	Sensitivity (%)	Specificity (%)	Unable to evaluate (%)
4 Slice	83	93	22
8 Slice	82	93	24
16 Slice	88	97	9
64 Slice	93	97	4

* Callister, The Tennessee Heart and Vascular Institute, unpublished written communication, November 4, 2005.

As the number of detector rows increases, the sensitivity and specificity of cardiac CTA levels off. However, with the 16- and 64-slice CT scanners, the number of uninterpretable scans markedly decreases because of the improved temporal and spatial resolution of these newer scanners.

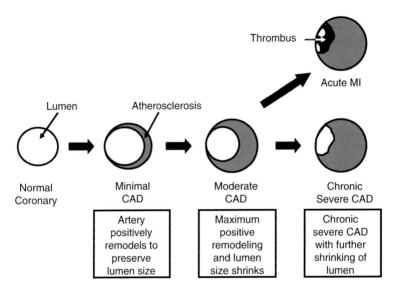

Figure 4.2. The Glagov phenomenon depicts the effect of positive remodeling on lumen size. As the extent of atherosclerosis increases, the lumen size may remain relatively unchanged until maximum positive remodeling occurs (relatively late in the disease process). Therefore, traditional diagnostic tests such as cardiac catheterization (lumen gram) may underestimate the extent of atherosclerosis, emphasizing the importance of testing such as cardiac CTA.

CTA is a wonderful technique to make the diagnosis of coronary artery disease because it is very sensitive in picking up soft plaque. Soft-plaque recognition will redefine a person's risk category. Almost 50% of low-risk-group patients have plaque by CTA and may, therefore, be treated more aggressively. Angiography is not better than CTA or vice versa. These techniques are just different and do different things. Therefore, the question asked needs to be understood and the two techniques need to be used to answer the specific questions for which they are best suited. Each test has its strengths and weaknesses. Cardiac catheterization is a representation of the coronary lumen only and does not account for the Glagov effect (positive remodeling to preserve the lumen size in early atherosclerosis) (Figure 4.2). Therefore, it may underestimate plaque burden.

Nuclear cardiology is limited in that it can only diagnose flow-limiting stenoses and can only rarely diagnose other causes of chest pain. Despite the above limitations, a normal nuclear stress test is associated with less than a 1% annual risk of a cardiac event. Most myocardial infarctions, however, are caused by low-grade stenoses.[17A] For this reason, the diagnosis of early cornary artery disease is critical and for this application cardiac CTA is well suited.

Figure 4.3 and Tables 4.2 and 4.3 list the sensitivity, specificity, and negative predictive power of cardiac CTA. The basic concept is to recognize the excellent negative predictive value of cardiac CTA. Most recently, one of the

Table 4.2. Multidetector computed tomography coronary angiography: initial results with 16-slice systems

Author	N	Sensitivity	Specificity	PPV	Lesions detected	Threshold
Cury[35]	58	95	80	80	82/86	>2 mm
Achenbach[36]	77	92	79	79	57/62	>1.5 mm
Keuttner[37]	57	74	71	71	51/69	None
Mollet[38]	128	92	80	80	216/234	>2 mm

PPV, positive predictive value; NPV, negative predictive value.

Table 4.3. Multidetector computed tomography coronary angiography: initial results with 64-slice systems

Author	No. of Patients ≠ segments	Patient type	Analysis by segment			Analysis by patient		
			Sensitivity	Specificity	PPV	Sensitivity	Specificity	PPV
Leber[39]	55/798	Stable angina	73	97	NR	88	85	NR
Leschka[40]	67/1005	Suspected CAD	94	97	87	100	100	100
Raff[41]	70/1065	Suspected CAD	86	95	66	95	90	93
Pugliese[42]	35/494	Stable angina	99	96	78	100	90	96

PPV, positive predictive value; NPV, negative predictive value; NR, not reported; CAD, coronary artery disease.

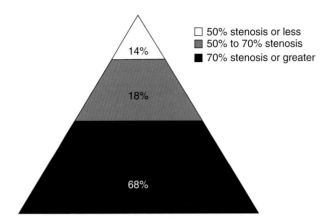

Figure 4.3. Coronary stenosis severity before myocardial infarction. The figure illustrates that most myocardial infarctions occur because of lesions of less than 50%. Thus, early detection of subclinical disease is crucial. (Ambrose et al. Circulation 1995.[17A])

first multicenter cardiac CTA studies assessed 187 patients with 16-slice CTA to determine the sensitivity and specificity to detect greater than 50% stenosis with angiographic correlation in all. This study found a sensitivity of 89% and a specificity of 63%.[18] The negative predictive value was still near 100%. Although this real-world multicenter trial yielded less impressive results than previous data suggest, better accuracy may be expected when this type of study is repeated with a 64-slice scanner.

5. Basic Concepts in Cardiac CTA

The CT Scanner (X-Ray Beam Production)

The cone shaped X-ray beams emanate from a source in the computed tomography (CT) gantry and terminate at the detectors on the other side of a rotating gantry. Each row of detectors is called a "channel" and each channel produces an image "slice." The Siemens scanner "wobbles" along the z-axis focal spot so that 32 channels produce 64 slices ("flying z spot"). In this way, an equivalent 64-slice scanner can be produced with only 32 detector rows or channels. More detector rows mean more radiation exposure.

The CT image is an overall estimate of the attenuation of the X-rays as they pass through the body (how many beams get through the body). This process creates an estimate of the computerized densities of the object through which the beams pass, acting like a density spectroscope, measuring the densities in three dimensions and displaying them on a computer screen. These densities are represented by Hounsfield units (discussed below). Projections in a 360-degree rotation of the scanner are collected in a computerized bin to narrow in on the true X-ray density and location of the object within the body. If enough projections are collected, a good estimate of the object's density and location can be created (Figure 5.1).

Figure 5.2 depicts a typical CT scanner setup. The concept is that the X-ray source and the detectors rotate (helical scanning technique) quickly around the gantry as the table moves through the gantry at a certain speed known as the pitch (described below). The breakthrough that has allowed rapid helical scanning is the slip ring. The slip ring allows data to be transferred from the detectors to the data assembly system (DAS) without the use of wires (*see* page 34).

The distance the table moves through the gantry in total defines the scan field. After determining the structures of interest, the technologist selects the scan field from the scout film or from the noncontrasted calcium score (CaSc) scan.

If the gantry rotates a full circle around the patient, a 360-degree image along the entire scan field is created. With a single-source CT scanner, the minimum gantry rotation necessary to provide a full circle image is 180 degrees (half-gantry rotation). With half-gantry rotation, the center point density of the object being imaged can be isolated by back calculating the remaining 180 degrees of the image. This reduced scan angle increases the temporal resolution of the scan.

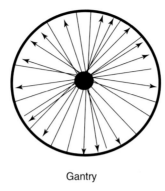

Gantry

Figure 5.1. X-ray beams emanating from a source rotating 360 degrees around the gantry. In reality, only a 180° rotation (1/2 gantry rotation) is employed. When enough attenuated X-ray beams reach the detector, the computer begins to localize the object of interest (in this case the black circle) and it also begins to narrow in on the estimate of the object's density.

The detected attenuated X-ray signal is converted to a raw dataset by the detectors via an electrical signal. This step requires a complex set of mathematical calculations. The raw data represent the acquired density measurements in the axial plane or *x-y*-axis. Reconstruction algorithms are then

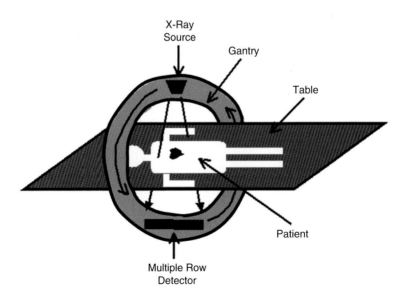

Figure 5.2. The typical single-source CT scanner in cartoon format.

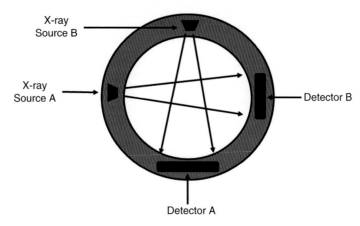

X-ray
Source B

X-ray
Source A

Detector B

Detector A

Figure 5.3. A typical dual-source CT scanner in which detector B must be smaller than detector A because of limits on space within the gantry.

performed on the raw data to estimate each projection line in an x- and y-axis, providing a precise three-dimensional location of a density within the body. This scan can also be gated to allow the object to be imaged at a specific point in the cardiac cycle.

The three-dimensional information and time information from each projection are collected into a mathematical gating bin. The raw data in this bin are then converted to a computerized image, which is viewed at the workstation. This image is a collection of all the density measurements at the various three-dimensional locations. The density measurements are scaled in Hounsfield units, which represent the degree of X-ray attenuation and are highly specific for various tissues and substances (discussed below).

The most frequently used scanners today have 64 rows or channels of detectors (i.e., 64-slice CT scanner) and one source of X-rays. Recent technological advancements have allowed the creation of a dual-source CT scanner (DSCT) with two X-ray sources and two sets of detectors as depicted in Figure 5.3. DSCT decreases the time to acquire one image slice because only 1/4 a gantry rotation is now required (quarter-gantry rotation), further improving the temporal resolution.

One detector (A) covers the entire scan field of view with a diameter of 50 cm whereas the other detector (B) is restricted to a smaller central field of view because of space limitations within the gantry. Because DSCT only requires 1/4 of a gantry rotation to complete a 360-degree image, the temporal resolution of a DSCT scanner is 83 ms without the need for multisegmental reconstruction techniques. With dual-segment reconstruction, the mean temporal resolution is 60 ms with a minimum temporal resolution 42 ms. The z flying focal spot technique implemented in the DSCT system produces a spatial resolution of 0.4 mm at all heart rates.[19]

X-Ray Detectors (X-Ray Beam Detection)

The CT detectors collect the attenuated X-ray beams as they pass through the patient. The temporal resolution of the image improves as the number of detector rows increases (4-, 8-, 16-, and 64-detector CT). Current standards demand at least 16 rows of detectors for an adequate diagnostic computed tomographic angiography (CTA) scan. Before the 16-slice scanners (4- and 8-slice), the temporal resolution of cardiac CTA was inadequate for consistent, diagnostic quality imaging of the coronary arteries.

Sixty-four-slice scanners are generally more accurate than 16-slice scanners.[20] A higher level of experience (technologist and cardiologist/radiologist alike) is necessary for successful with a 16-slice scanner. A 16-slice scanner can be differentiated from a 64-slice scanner by the width of the image slabs (Figure 5.4). The 64-slice scanner has wider image slabs because the coverage area per gantry rotation is greater (28 to 40 mm).

In addition, with the 16-slice scanner, a longer scan time is necessary, and therefore, there is a greater likelihood that motion artifacts caused by breathing, increased heart rate, or heart rate variability will interfere with the scan quality. From 4- to 8- to 16- to 64-slice systems, the breath hold time for helical scanning of the heart has been significantly reduced. However, it is only with the 256-slice system that the entire heart can be scanned with one single gantry rotation.

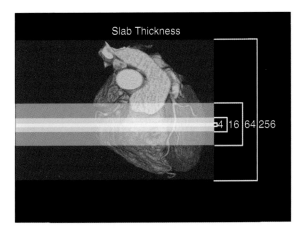

Figure 5.4. As the detector row number increases from 4 to 8 to 16 to 64 to 256, the slab thickness increases as well. Increased slab thicknesses translate to less gantry rotations necessary for complete imaging of the heart. The fewer gantry rotations required, the shorter the scan time (i.e., less heart beats and shorter breath hold). Only the 256-detector scanners can accomplish complete cardiac coverage in one gantry rotation.

Resolution

There are three types of resolution to consider: spatial resolution, temporal resolution, and contrast resolution. The spatial resolution is defined as the narrowest distance between which two objects may be discriminated. Objects further apart than the spatial resolution limits should be distinguishable. Essentially, one is interested in both the in-plane spatial resolution (x-, y-axis) and the through-plane spatial resolution (z-axis).

The in-plane resolution is determined by the geometric characteristics of the scanners and the through-plane resolution is determined by the collimator width. Currently, the CT machines have reached maximum resolution in these two areas because the individual detector cannot physically be made smaller at this time and the geometric characteristics of the scanners are optimized. In addition, the collimator width cannot be decreased because by doing so, excess radiation would be required to allow adequate imaging.

The through-plane resolution defines the axial slice thickness. The narrower the slice thickness, the more necessary radiation because narrower slice thicknesses create more noise and more energy is necessary to overcome the noise. The axial spatial resolution is related to the width of the detectors in the detectors array where the center of the detector array has better spatial through-plane resolution than the outer sections of the detector array. CTA does not yet have adequate spatial resolution to grade the percent stenosis as specifically as we do with angiography.

The temporal resolution is defined as the frequency with which an object is imaged or the time increment between successive images. In the case of cardiac CTA, this would represent the ability to accurately image the heart independent of its motion, or in other words, the ability of the scanner to freeze cardiac motion for purposes of imaging. The technological breakthrough that improved the temporal resolution of cardiac CTA to allow diagnostic coronary evaluations was the slip ring, which allows data to be transferred from the detectors to the DAS without wires. This permits helical scanning where the gantry rotates freely and continuously to provide a constant stream of X-rays for the purpose of providing the most imaging data in the shortest possible time. If wires were necessary, the gantry would not be able to rotate quickly and continuously because the wires would tangle. The slip ring negates the need for connecting wires between the detectors and the DAS.

Contrast resolution is the ability to distinguish objects of similar density. Below is a list of the various resolution types of multiple common cardiac imaging modalities.

1. Cardiac catheterization spatial resolution = 0.2 mm
2. Cardiac catheterization temporal resolution = 33 frames per second or approximately 8 ms
3. Single photon emission CT (SPECT) spatial resolution = 7–14 mm
4. SPECT temporal resolution: only uses eight phases within each R-R interval
5. SPECT contrast resolution: 40%–60% of patients have attenuation

6. Positron emission tomography (PET) spatial resolution = 7 mm
7. Echo spatial resolution = 1 mm
8. Echo temporal resolution = 33 ms or better with digital.
9. Echo contrast resolution: 25%–40% will have suboptimal studies
10. Magnetic resonance imaging (MRI) spatial resolution: 0.5–1 mm.
11. CTA spatial resolution = 0.4 mm in the x- and y-axis and to 0.6 mm in the z-axis (slice thickness).
12. CTA temporal resolution = 60–220 ms depending on the vendor and reconstruction type used.
13. Intravascular ultrasound (IVUS) spatial resolution = 0.5–0.8 mm.

In summary, with regard to temporal and spatial resolution, catheterization is better than CTA, which is better than magnetic resonance angiography (MRA). In the case of contrast resolution, CTA is better than MRA, which is better than catheterization. As far as radiation dose, MRA uses less radiation than catheterization, which in turn uses less radiation than CTA. For morphology and plaque assessment, IVUS is better than CTA, which is better than MRA, which is better than catheterization.

Collimators

Emitted X-ray beams must pass through the collimator before reaching the patient and subsequently the detectors. Collimators shape or "collimate" the X-ray beam to a certain width. The collimators help to control the width of the emitted X-ray beam, the detector configuration used to sense the emitted X-rays, and the quality and position of the X-ray beams. In addition, the collimators help to protect the patient by filtering the emitted X-rays and by controlling the amount of scatter. These functions aid the CT scanner in accurately detecting the exact location from which the detected X-rays emanated. By doing this, structures are then positioned accurately in the image. Finally, as stated above, the collimators help to determine the through-plane (z-axis) spatial resolution or slice thickness (amount of territory covered with one gantry rotation). The term collimator differs from the term collimation which is defined as a product of the detector number and the slice thickness.

At the present time, the effective collimator width is the width of the detectors themselves. Essentially this means there is no space between individual detectors. In addition, there is no space between detector rows. Therefore, the minimum collimator width cannot be improved upon unless the physical width of a detector is narrowed. With the 64-slice scanner, each detector is 0.6 mm thick and thus the collimator width is effectively 0.6 mm. Therefore, the narrowest slice thickness is approximately 0.6 mm (z-plane resolution). With mathematical manipulation, this limit may be improved to 0.4 mm. At the present time, the collimator width cannot be decreased and thus 0.4 mm is currently the best achievable through-plane (z-axis) resolution.

The collimator width does not affect the in-plane (x-, y-axis) spatial resolution, which is 0.6 mm as well. This limit is defined by the inherent geometric characteristics of the scanner. At the present time, the limitations of physics do not allow the detector row thickness to decrease and thus the geometric characteristics of the CT scanner are presently optimized to the maximum and thus 0.6 mm is currently the best achievable x-, y-plane spatial resolution.

It should be also be noted that temporal resolution is also unaffected by the collimator width because it is defined by the gantry rotation speed. Presently, the maximum gantry rotation speed is 330 ms (Siemens scanner). With half-gantry rotation, the effective temporal resolution improves to 165 ms. Multisegment reconstruction (recognizing its limitations) will maximize temporal resolution to approximately 85 ms.

Contrast resolution is defined as the ability to distinguish objects of different contrast densities and will also remain unchanged by the collimator width. Current CT scanners have excellent contrast resolution.

Finally, the volume of coverage (Slab Thickness, Figure 5.4) of each gantry rotation is defined by the detector array number. With the 64-detector row CT machine, there is 28–40 mm of territory covered with each gantry rotation. The exact-slab thickness is vendor specific and depends on the slice thickness. For a 64-slice scanner with a slice thickness of 0.625 mm the slab thickness is 40 mm ($0.625 \times 64 = 40$), meaning that each slab of data will then be approximately 40 mm thick. The average coverage necessary for the heart (scan field) is 120 mm, so generally, in this example, there will be three slabs needed to cover the entire heart with the 64-detector scanners ($40 \times 3 = 120$). With the 16 detector row scanners, there is approximately 7–10 mm of coverage with each gantry rotation resulting in a slab thickness of 7–10 mm. Therefore, with a 16-slice scanner, more slabs are necessary to cover the entire heart. One way to determine which CT scanner (16- versus 64-slice) was used to generate an image is to check the slab thickness on the image. The image with the thicker slabs is the one created by the 64-slice scanner.

The soon to be developed 256-detector scanners will improve the volume of coverage to include the entire heart in one beat thereby decreasing the scan time and breath hold time. The 256-slice scanners will also eliminate problems from heart rate variability because only one beat is required to image the heart. However, resolution will not change because the collimator width, geometric characteristics of the scanner, and the gantry rotation speed will not change. Note that as the detector array number increases, gantry weight will increase thereby potentially decreasing the gantry rotation time. Thus, with a greater detector array number, the temporal resolution may theoretically decrease. Further studies are necessary to determine if the 256-slice scanners will effectively be an improvement over the current 64-slice scanners.

To create the entire cardiac CTA image, all the slabs are stacked together and recreated into a single image like a stack of books. All slabs should line up nicely when reconstructed. Failure of the slabs to line up correctly represents misregistration, which is discussed below.

Computer Screen Matrix

The matrix of the computer screen defines the number of pixels or voxels within the screen. In CTA, the computer screen matrix size is 512×512 (Figure 5.5). In MRI, the matrix size is usually only 256×256. Therefore, CT scanning

Each square dot represents 1 individual pixel that is 13 volume units deep into the screen creating a 3-dimensional pixel which in turn is called a voxel. In this example, the matrix is 18 voxels by 12 voxels. The true CTA matrix is 512 voxels by 512 voxels. By assigning a gray scale value to each individual volume unit (13 in this example), a greater possible number of shades of gray may then be potentially depicted onto the computer screen. An isotropic voxel is one where the spatial resolution is equal in all 3 planes. Isotropic voxels are what allow 3-D volume rendered images.

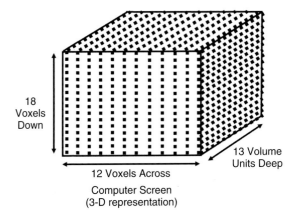

18
Voxels
Down

13 Volume
Units Deep

12 Voxels Across

Computer Screen
(3-D representation)

Figure 5.5. Cartoon depiction of the computer screen matrix.

is better than MRI in this regard because it offers more data points per image and, thus, better resolution.

Windowing

Windowing is a term used for fine adjustments made to the image to enhance viewing and to emphasize various structures of interest (tweaking the image to pick up detail).

Hounsfield units measure how much the X-rays are attenuated. In other words, Hounsfield units are used to describe the brightness of an object when the object is represented on the computer screen. It is a scale created to estimate the degree of absorption of the X-ray beam as it passes through the body and is subsequently received by the detector array. This scale allows objects of different densities to be displayed differently on the computer screen. More dense objects are brighter than less dense objects when using the Hounsfield unit scale (see below).

The CT machine is calibrated and balanced daily so that the furthest left on the Hounsfield unit scale is the least dense and is calibrated to air and assigned absolute black. The middle of the scale is assigned 0 and a middle-gray color. This middle gray represents the water density of which the body is primarily composed.

Because the human eye cannot distinguish between the 5000–10,000 possible shades of gray, the gray scale must be compressed to approximately 500 different shades, which is the maximum number appreciated by the human eye. This process is called windowing and the number of shades of gray in the compressed scale is called the window width (WW). The WW is the scaled-down compression of the gray scale range (to around 500 from the total of nearly 5000–10,000) when going from black to white. In other words, the number of possible shades of gray must be compressed to optimize viewing by the human eye. The selected WW artificially defines this number. Therefore, 90% of the viewing information is effectively discarded when a WW is selected.

The window level (WL) is defined as the centerline of the WW. That is, the WL defines where the WW is located along the entire Hounsfield unit scale. The WL is adjusted along the Hounsfield unit scale to focus viewing on various tissues and structures. Everything to the left of the WL is black and everything to the right of the WL is white (Figures 5.6 and 5.7). Remember the Hounsfield unit measurement is a Gaussian curve representing the true density of the object.

Poon has described that the best WW and WL for diagnosing coronary artery disease is 700 and 350, respectively (M. Poon, Cabrini Medical Center, New York, NY, unpublished oral communication, February 6, 2006).

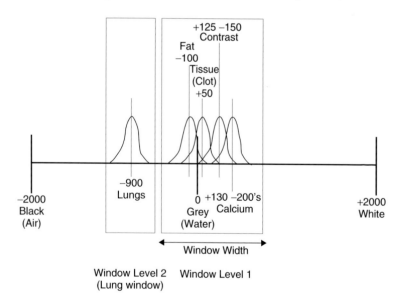

Figure 5.6. The Hounsfield scale. In particular, the WW and WL are depicted in cartoon format.

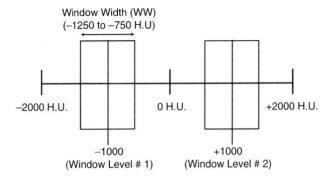

Window Level (WL) is the Center line of Window Width (WW)

Figure 5.7. Two separate windows with similar WWs. The WL of each separate window is the center line density of each WW. H.U., Hounsfield units.

Hounsfield Unit Measurements

- Atheroma (soft plaque) = +20 to +130 (average approximately +70)
- Soft plaque ≅ +50
- Calcified plaque = +130–200. Plaque characterization beyond calcified or "soft" is not yet ready for prime time. However, recently reported data indicate that intraplaque enhancement corresponds with neovascularization of the plaque (portraying an increased risk for intraplaque hemorrhage) and implies an unstable lesion.[21]
- Contrast = ≥ +125 to 300 to 400
- Thrombus = +50
- Tissue = +50
- Blood = +30
- Gadolinium = +50
- Calcium without contrast present = +130–200's
- Calcium with contrast present = +350–400 (high amounts of contrast can overwhelm the calcium. Remember, calcium formation is a gradual process and the density may vary with the age of the calcium.
- Fat = −80 to −100
- Air = −900 to −1000
- Beam hardening artifact ≤ −50
- Water (fluid or cysts) = −20 to +20

Field of View

Field of view (FOV) may be described in terms of the selected FOV (sFOV) and the displayed FOV (dFOV). The sFOV is the chosen area or region within the body that one wishes to reconstruct and transfer to the workstation. In other words, the sFOV is the box of data chosen from the entire scanned raw data to be reconstructed. The dFOV is the portion of the sFOV that is actually displayed on the 512×512 computer screen matrix. If the dFOV visualized on the screen at the workstation differs from the sFOV, then a digital zoom has occurred. The image has thus been digitally magnified.

The sFOV is divided by the matrix size to yield the number of pixels that will be needed to display the image. The smaller the sFOV (chosen region of interest) displayed on the screen, the larger the image will appear on the screen. This increases the spatial resolution by increasing the number of voxels per millimeter of the picture, thus maximizing the information or data per voxel. Therefore, by making the sFOV smaller, resolution will inherently be increased.

When doing cardiac CTA, always use the smallest sFOV possible to increase the spatial resolution to the maximum. Do not give away resolution by increasing the sFOV more than necessary to include the structures of interest. Excellent spatial resolution is required to evaluate the coronary arteries. Thus, if concerned about only the coronaries, choose a sFOV that covers only the heart and no more. In addition, the smaller the sFOV, the less the liability for areas not visualized with regard to noncardiac findings.

After reconstructing the chosen sFOV, one can digitally zoom the displayed image on the computer screen at the workstation to decrease the dFOV and make a smaller structure appear larger on the screen (zoom in on a structure). However, in general, the integrity of the image breaks down if the image is zoomed more than 1 or 2 times. So, the sFOV is the key.

Most hearts fit into a 15- to 17-cm sFOV. Most technologists are trained to choose an sFOV of 25 cm. As the technologist gets more comfortable, train them to reduce the sFOV to 15–17 cm to include only the heart and superiorly to the bifurcation of the pulmonary artery. The sFOV may be widened just a little bit to accommodate translation of the heart during the scan. In theory, the sFOV can be reduced even more to include only a small portion of the heart such as the left main coronary artery if the left main is the only structure of interest. This type of sFOV would be done in only rare incidences such as the assessment of a questionable angiographic finding.

Remember, the actual raw data will include a much larger region than the sFOV. By narrowing the sFOV, the technologist has requested to reconstruct only a small portion of the raw data and has chosen to display only this portion on the workstation. In other words, the scan encompasses all of the raw data included in the scan volume, but the technologist gives instructions to the computer to reconstruct around only the center point of the requested sFOV. Once this is done, the center of the image cannot be changed. Before discarding the raw data, different sFOV reconstructions can be obtained if needed. After discarding the raw data (too large of a dataset to store indefinitely), one cannot go back to the raw dataset.

Pitch

The pitch is essentially the speed of the table as it moves through the gantry. The table feed is defined as the distance the table moves through the gantry in one gantry rotation. The pitch is defined as the table feed divided by the collimator width. The pitch may be varied with some scanners but it is fixed in other scanners such as the Siemens. In general, the average pitch is 10 mm of table advancement per rotation, divided by the slab thickness of 40 mm in the Siemens 64-slice scanner, which yields a usual pitch of about 0.25.

A pitch of 0.25 will create a twenty-five percent overlap of data among the various slabs. This overlap is necessary because it creates an important redundancy of data, which is necessary because not all of the data occurs in the most opportune time in the cardiac cycle. Data collected at inopportune times within the cardiac cycle will be less reliable. Image slabs are thus overlapped to duplicate data, increasing confidence in the validity of the image by building in a redundancy of data. In general, a pitch of 1 will create no overlap and no gaps between slabs. A pitch of greater than 1 will leave gaps between slabs and a pitch of less than 1 will allow the necessary overlap among slabs.

Triggering

Two types of triggering or electrocardiogram (ECG) gating exist: prospective (Figure 5.8) and retrospective (Figure 5.9).

Prospective triggering is where the scanner emits radiation only at a predefined point after the R wave (a constant cardiac phase). At all other times between each R-R interval or at all other cardiac phases, the CTA machine is shut off and no radiation is emitted. This triggering method requires a regular heart rate or the image created during each heartbeat will occur at different cardiac phases, resulting in significant misregistration artifacts. Prospective triggering also requires very thick collimators, which will not suffice to sufficiently examine the coronary arteries. Therefore, at this time, prospective triggering is only used for calcium scoring.

Calcium scoring can also be done with retrospective triggering but this is not advised because retrospective triggering requires more radiation. Prospective triggering reduces the radiation dose by up to 10 times, but occurs at a cost in that it does not allow the reader to change phases during image analysis because it is not a continuous scan. With the newest 256-slice scanners, prospective triggering may become useful for CTA because the heart can be imaged in one beat because of the increased coverage per gantry rotation. The 256-slice scanners also increase the temporal resolution, allowing successful imaging at increased heart rates. But remember, with increased heart rates, dose modulation (discussed on page 44) cannot be used, thus increasing radiation exposure. The proper imaging techniques are at this time changing rapidly and continuing to improve.

Retrospective triggering is the most frequently used method for cardiac CTA at this time. Here, a continuous heart scan is utilized (throughout the entire cardiac cycle). After the scan, a specific cardiac phase (point within the R-R interval) is retrospectively chosen to create image stacks. In this case, there is a true match of the data to the ECG, allowing coverage through the entire cardiac cycle. There are two techniques to retrospectively gate the scan to the ECG for image reconstruction. In the first method, image stacks from each heartbeat are collected at a specified time within the cardiac cycle defined as the percent of the R-R interval. The second method is to choose an absolute fixed time in milliseconds before or after the R wave in order to reconstruct image sets for each separate heartbeat. This method is better if the heart rhythm is irregular. To maximize the likelihood of a diagnostic dataset, the electrocardiographic data from the scan duration should be previewed before selecting which retrospective gating technique to use.

Retrospective triggering permits faster coverage of the heart than does prospective triggering because stacks of images are reconstructed at every heartbeat. Continuous spiral acquisition allows overlapping of image sections

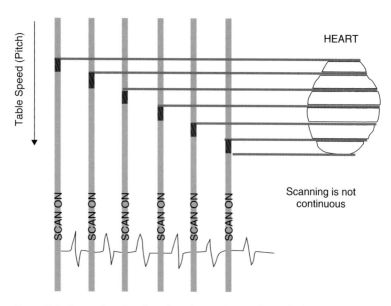

Figure 5.8. Prospective triggering where the scan is turned on only during a preselected point within the cardiac cycle and no radiation is emitted between these points. Depending on the heart rate, different numbers of heartbeats are required to completely reconstruct an entire image of the heart. This triggering method permits only one cardiac phase to be imaged but uses markedly reduced amounts of radiation.

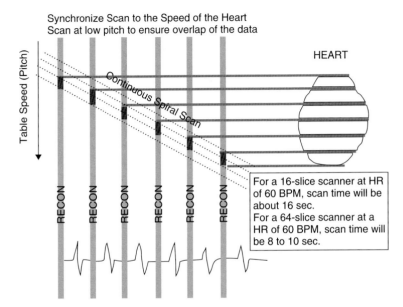

Figure 5.9. Retrospective triggering where the radiation is continuously emitted throughout the entire cardiac cycle. A discrete time between each R-R interval is retrospectively chosen for image reconstruction (Recon). This triggering method allows the operator to reconstruct an image at any selected point within the R-R interval at a cost of more emitted radiation.

and therefore results in 20% greater in-plane spatial resolution than that allowed by the collimator itself, resulting in a resolution of 0.6 mm for a 0.75-mm section and 0.4 mm for a 0.6-mm section. Therefore, retrospective triggering is the preferred method of triggering for imaging the coronary arteries and heart structures.

Continuous acquisition throughout the cardiac cycle also allows retrospective reconstruction at different phases of the cardiac cycle to optimize the image in the face of intrinsic cardiac motion. The optimal phase may be different for certain structures such as the right coronary artery (RCA), which demonstrates the most motion throughout the cardiac cycle. Finally, individual heartbeats may be deleted after the fact or the reconstruction interval for an individual beat can be shifted manually if needed. Electrocardiographic editing, however, may not be available on all systems.

Proper ECG lead placement is also important to assure a good tracing. Keep the wires away from the heart so as not to create artifacts in the image (windmill artifact).

Radiation

The X-ray dose is determined by the X-ray tube voltage in KVp and the tube current in milliamperes (mA). The KVp choices are generally 80, 100, 120 or 140 but are rarely altered from the recommended settings. The milliamperes per second (mAs) is the tube current unit reported in most CT machines and is defined as the product of the mA and the gantry rotation time in seconds. The effective tube current (effective mAs) is the product of the mAs and the pitch.

Center beam collimation and more detector rows generally increases radiation dose. In addition, the slower the pitch the more total radiation delivered throughout the scan because the patient is under the scanner for a longer period of time. The level of radiation for gated spiral CTA of the heart is contributed by continuous overlapping data acquisition at a highly overlapping spiral pitch.

The radiation dose should always be minimized whenever possible. Dose modulation or ECG pulsing (Figure 5.10) is used to help reduce the radiation exposure. With dose modulation, the radiation level is reduced by 40%–50%. Dose modulation is a method in which the mA is dialed down by 80% during systole. In dose modulation mode, the highest mA is present only during 40%–80% of the R-R interval and the radiation dose is reduced by 40%. However, when this technique is used, the rhythm must be stable and the heart rate must be slow. If not, the systolic phases will contain images too poor for diagnostic purposes in the multiphasic analysis because the systolic radiation dose is too low during dose modulation. With most machines, dose modulation is the default mode and needs to be turned off if its use is not desired. If the heart rate is ≥75 bpm, do not use dose modulation because it becomes

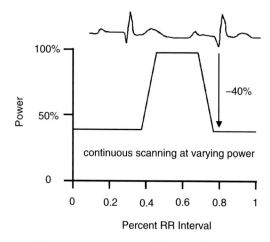

Figure 5.10. Graphic illustration of the concept of ECG pulsing (dose modulation). The power is selectively increased at predefined points within the cardiac cycle to reduce the overall radiation exposure during the scan.

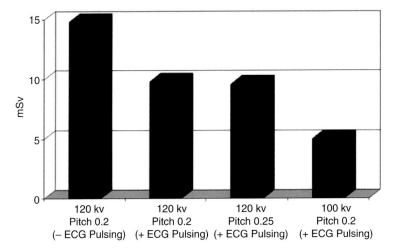

Figure 5.11. Patient exposure dose in millisieverts for various scanning protocols; estimates for coronary 64-slice CT angiography. Patient radiation exposure depends heavily on the imaging protocol type.

more likely that the systolic phases will be needed for analysis. At this reduced power, the systolic phases are still adequate for gated motion analysis applications.

In addition to ECG pulsing, one can minimize the sFOV to reduce the patient's time under the scanner, thus reducing the patient's total radiation exposure. Imaging protocols can have substantial effect on radiation dose (Figure 5.11).[22]

Definitions

Radiation energy is the number of protons pushed.

Effective dose (E): Reflects the nonuniform radiation absorption of partial body exposure relative to whole body radiation. E is calculated from information about dose to an individual organ and is expressed in millisieverts (mSv) or sieverts (Sv). E is weighted in terms of relative risk to a particular body region.

Radiation Units: $E = k$ (constant, Table 5.1) $\times$ DLP (dose length product)
1 millicurie (mCi) = 37 millibecquerels (mBq)
1 rad = 1 rem (for X-rays and gamma rays). A rad is the radiation dose divided by 1 cm^3 of tissue.
100 rad = 1 gray (Gy)
100 rem = 1 Sv

Table 5.1. The k, DLP, and E for various body parts

	k	DLP	E
Head	0.0023	790	1.8
Neck	0.0054	250	1.3
Chest	0.017	450	7.7
Abdomen	0.015	600	9
Pelvis	0.019	650	12

DLP: The amount of radiation absorbed in the body, which is an indication of the integrated radiation dosage of an entire CT examination. It incorporates the number of scans and the length of the scan.

$$DLP = CTDI_{vol} \times \text{scan length}$$
(See below for an explanation of $CTDI_{vol}$.)

$$mSv = DLP \times k$$

What is k? k is a constant that differs for different parts of the body (Table 5.1).

$$k = (mSv \times mGy^{-1} \times cm^{-1})$$

Example: How much radiation from a CTA to the chest does a patient receive if the total DLP is 1000?

$$mSv = DLP \times k$$
$$mSv = 0.017 \times 1000$$
$$= 17 \text{ mSv}$$

Ways to lower the DLP include using smaller scan lengths, excluding the CaSc, limiting the number of images, slowing the heart rate, or using dose modulation (ECG pulsing).

Radiation exposure: Number of ionizing events in the air.

Radiation dose or absorbed radiation dose: Amount of radiation energy deposited in the body from exposure.

CTDI: Absorbed dose measured by thermoluminescent dosimeter. It represents the integral under the radiation dose profile in the z-axis and depends on scan length.

$CTDI_{100}$ (coulomb/kg or C/kg): Convenient measure of exposure, which integrates the radiation exposure of a single scan over a length of 100 mm.

$CTDI_w$: A weighted average of the $CTDI_{100}$ measurements at the center and the peripheral locations of the phantom. It reflects the average absorbed dose over the x and y dimensions and approximates the average radiation dose to a cross-section of the patient's body.

$CTDI_{vol}$: A new radiation dose parameter and the preferred expression of CT dosimetry. It represents the average radiation dose over the x-, y-, and z-planes.

$$CTDI_{vol} = 1/\text{pitch} \times CTDI_w$$

Radiation dosage of selected exposures[22A]:
Posterior-anterior (PA) chest X-ray (CXR): 0.02 mSv. Therefore, 20 mSv
    is 1000 CXRs
PA and lateral CXR: 0.08 mSv
Mammogram: 0.13 mSv
Average USA background radiation: 3.0 mSv/year
Smoking cigarettes: 2.8 mSv/year
Air travel: 0.01 mSv/1000 miles

Estimated risk of 10-mSv dose of radiation:
1 in 1000 extra lifetime risk of cancer[23]
1 in 2000 extra risk of fatal cancer[23]

Radiation dosage of selected cardiovascular studies (total body effective
dose):
Multidetector CT (MDCT) coronary calcium scoring in a male (no dose
    modulation): 2.3–2.9 mSv
MDCT coronary calcium scoring in a male (with dose modulation):
    1.3–1.4 mSv
16-Slice MDCT coronary CTA in a male (no dose modulation):
    7.9–11.8 mSv
16-Slice MDCT coronary CTA in a male (with dose modulation):
    4.0–6.2 mSv
64-Slice MDCT coronary CTA in a male (no dose modulation):
    9.6–15.2 mSv
64-Slice MDCT coronary CTA in a male (with dose modulation):
    4.8–10 mSv
MDCT coronary calcium scoring in a female (no dose modulation): 3.2
    to 3.6 mSv
MDCT coronary calcium scoring in a female (with dose modulation):
    1.9–2.0 mSv
16-Slice MDCT coronary CTA in a female (no dose modulation):
    11.1–16.3 mSv
16-Slice MDCT coronary CTA in a female (with dose modulation):
    5.6–8.7 mSv
64-Slice MDCT coronary CTA in a female (no dose modulation):
    13.5–21.4 mSv
64-Slice MDCT coronary CTA in a female (with dose modulation):
    6.8–14 mSv
Tc-99m tetrofosmin rest-stress (10 mCi + 30 mCi): 10.6 mSv
Tc-99m sestamibi 1-day rest-stress (10 mCi + 30 mCi): 12 mSv
Tc-99m sestamibi 2-day stress-rest (30 mCi + 30 mCi): 17.5 mSv
Tl-201 stress and reinjection (3.0 mCi + 1.0 mCi): 25.1 mSv
Dual-isotope (3.0 mCi Tl-201 + 30 mCi Tc-99m): 27.3 mSv
Rb-82 PET myocardial perfusion (45 mCi + 45 mCi): 16 mSv
Ge-68 transmission for PET: 0.08 mSv
Gd-153 transmission for SPECT: 0.05 mSv
Cs-137 transmission for PET: 0.01 mSv
CT transmission source for PET (low-dose CT protocol): 0.8 mSv
Fluorine 18 fluorodeoxyglucose PET viability (10 mCi): 7 mSv

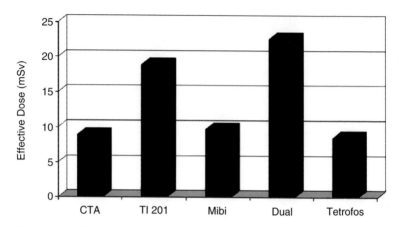

Figure 5.12. Effective radiation exposure dose for various cardiac imaging procedures. T1201, thallium 201; Mibi, sestamibi; Dual, dualisotope; Tetrofos, Tetrofosmin.

Radionuclide angiogram, Tc-99m-labeled red blood cells (20 mCi Tc-99m): 5.2 mSv

Iodine 123 MIBG myocardial imaging (10 mCi): 4.8 mSv

Iodine 123 BMIPP myocardial imaging (5 mCi): 4.7 mSv

Ventilation/perfusion lung (200 mBq Tc-99m MAA + 70 mBq Tc-99m aerosol): 2.8 mSv

Atrial fibrillation ablation: 12–14 mSv

Coronary angiogram: 2–3 mSv

Cardiac catheterization with left ventriculography: 6–8 mSv; cardiac catheterization with left ventriculogram is more than coronary angiogram alone because more energy is needed to penetrate the heart with all the contrast in it.

Nuclear stress tests can have more radiation exposure than cardiac CTA! If dose modulation is used, the radiation for a cardiac CTA can be one third that of a dual isotope nuclear scan. Figure 5.12[23] depicts radiation exposure for various cardiac procedures.

Ways to reduce radiation exposure include scanning for appropriate indications only, limiting the scan volume, reducing the heart rate, ECG dose modulation whenever possible, improved temporal and spatial resolution, more "efficient" imaging with improved detectors and sources, and prospective triggering.

Imaging Planes

Standard radiology imaging planes are related to the standard three-dimensional axes where the in-plane axes are the x-, y-axis or the left to right and back to front plane. The through-plane is the z-axis or the head to toe plane. The axial data (x-y-plane) is the original raw dataset and is the most pristine and least distorted orientation because it requires only one row of detectors at a time. In addition, the creation of the axial images requires no postprocessing.

The standard anatomic imaging planes used by the radiologist are the coronal view (front to back), the sagittal view (side to side), and the axial view (head to toe). However, these standard anatomic imaging planes are not appropriate for the heart, which does not sit in the body in a way that makes these views useful. Therefore, to make cardiac CT imaging more intuitive and practical, the images must be rotated to find appropriate views for cardiac anatomy. For cardiac structure, standard echocardiographic views may be created and for coronary imaging, angiographic views would be most useful. This approach may be named the cardiocentric approach (Callister, The Tennessee Heart and Vascular Institute. Unpublished oral communication, November 4, 2005).

The reader creates cardiocentric-imaging planes to make viewing the coronary arteries, and the cardiac structures themselves, more intuitive, and more comparable to those imaging modalities most familiar to the cardiologist (such as ECG and coronary angiography). An apical four-chamber echocardiographic view can be created and equates to the left anterior oblique (LAO) cranial angiographic view. This angle gives a great view of the mid-left anterior descending coronary artery (LAD) and posterior descending coronary artery (PDA) and is also good for the distal right coronary artery (RCA) branches. This is also the view that allows adequate analysis of the cardiac chambers.

An echocardiographically equivalent short-axis view will mimic the LAO caudal or spider angiographic view. This view will be excellent for the circumflex and its branches and will also allow very good visualization of the left main coronary artery. In addition, this view is great to identify myocardial bridges.

Finally, an image equivalent to the parasternal long-axis echocardiographic view mimics the angiographic right anterior oblique (RAO) caudal projection. This is a wonderful orientation for visualization of the distal circumflex and obtuse marginal arteries. In addition, this view is excellent for the RCA, the proximal LAD, and the left atrial appendage.

These views may be constructed and saved as presets in most workstations. Because each individual's heart is oriented differently in the body, slight adjustments must be made when analyzing patient-specific images despite the presets. Nevertheless, presets will certainly speed up the reading process. Navigating through the images is essential and demands a great deal of familiarity with the workstation and much practice.

6. Essentials in Creating a Diagnostic Cardiac CTA Image

The three general steps to successfully creating a cardiac computed tomographic angiography (CTA) image are described below and depicted in Figure 6.1 (Callister, The Tennessee Heart and Vascular Institute, unpublished written communication, November 4, 2005).

Data Acquisition

The data acquisition stage is when the raw data are collected as the patient is being scanned. This is the stage in which the X-rays emanate from the source as the gantry continuously rotates around the table. The X-rays are then detected by the detector rows and moved to the data acquisition system (DAS) through the slip ring and stored in a mathematical, computerized bin as raw axial data for later reconstruction.

Patient Selection

It is crucial to educate the referring doctors to pick appropriate patients for referral. In addition, it is equally important to instill confidence in the referring physicians and thus avoid promising more than the technique can deliver.

Diagnostic image quality is difficult to obtain in morbidly obese patients. Therefore, as a general rule, avoid CTA in patients with a body mass index greater than 40. However, exceptions exist and individual patients should be evaluated on a case-to-case basis. For example, if an obese patient carries most of his or her weight below the waist (pear shaped), adequate imaging of the chest may still be possible. In addition, if the clinical question is limited (i.e., left main coronary artery or pulmonary veins), a diagnostic CTA may still be obtained in these patients.

If a large patient is imaged, the mAs (power) must be increased. The usual mAs is approximately 750–800. The mAs may be increased to as high as 850 to even 950 in large patients to increase the signal-to-noise ratio. Thicker slices (0.75 mm) will also increase signal-to-noise ratio at the expense of less through-plane spatial resolution.

In addition, the iodine flux must be maximized in larger patients to increase contrast opacification. The iodine flux is related to the iodine concen-

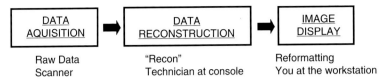

Figure 6.1. The necessary steps to creating a successful cardiac CTA image. "Recon", reconstruction.

tration and the bolus administration rate, and represents the key to obtaining adequate contrast opacification. Therefore, intracoronary contrast opacification may be improved in obese patients by increasing the iodine concentration or by increasing the rate of bolus administration. Iodine concentrations are generally listed as 320, 350, or 370 (i.e., Optiray 350) and bolus administration rates may vary from a high of 6 or 7 cc/second in the obese patient to 4 cc/second in the small patient. The usual bolus administration rate is 5 cc/second.

It should be noted that the iodine flux is also affected by uncontrollable variables such as cardiac output (the product of stroke volume and heart rate). Patients with diminished cardiac output may have inadequate contrast opacification despite optimization of the controllable variables mentioned above because the iodine flux will be diminished. Remember, ejection fraction is not equivalent to the cardiac output. Patients with diminished ejection fractions may still have adequate cardiac output for optimal contrast opacification.

Keep in mind that the total volume of contrast needed for a CTA is the product of the scan time and the contrast flow rate. Although the contrast volume does not determine the iodine flux, minimizing contrast is important to help reduce contrast toxicity.

CTA imaging of patients with extensive coronary calcification on the non-contrasted initial scan should also be avoided if possible. Extensive, diffuse coronary calcium will obscure visualization of the artery lumen, making diagnostic imaging near impossible. Some believe that if the calcium score (CaSc) is more than 1000, the CTA should be canceled. Exceptions would include focal areas of calcium that increase the total CaSc without diffusely obscuring visualization of the coronary lumen. It is not necessarily the amount of calcium that determines the adequacy of lumen visualization, but rather the location of the calcium (focal or diffuse). In addition, if particular clinical questions involve anatomic locations free of calcium, the CTA may still be useful.

Pacemakers do not preclude cardiac CTA. Usually, image quality is not significantly impaired. Interpretation, however, is more difficult in patients with implantable defibrillators (especially in interpreting the right coronary artery) and is virtually impossible in patients with biventricular pacing devices. CTA imaging of patients with biventricular pacemakers should be avoided, and limitations in interpretation should be accepted in patients with implantable defibrillators.

Avoid CTA imaging in patients with arrhythmias and markedly irregularly heart rhythms. Limited ectopy can be handled by electrocardiographic editing (if permitted by the specific scanner). Extensive electrocardiographic editing, however, will eliminate too much data for a full reconstruction and create banding artifacts or "holes" in the reconstructed image (see section on artifacts on page 85). These artifacts represent data loss.

Finally, at the present time, routine imaging of coronary stents should be avoided unless the stent is ≥3.5–4.0 mm. Certain stents are easily visualized by coronary CTA (Velocity stents) whereas others are not (Cypher stents). See page 104 for evaluation of stents.

Patient Preparation

The patient should be instructed to present to the scanning suite well hydrated. Taking nothing by mouth (NPO) may produce a state of dehydration, increasing the chance for tachycardia. Intravascular depletion also increases the risk for dye-induced nephrotoxicity and nitrate-induced tachycardia. In addition, when patients are NPO they tend to forget to take their medicines. Recommend no solids and no caffeine 12 hours before testing to avoid tachycardia. Clear liquid meals are recommended.

Instruct patients to take their medications as scheduled. Missing β-blocker doses, for example, will result in tachycardia and potential heart rate irregularity during the scan. In addition, advise patients to avoid significant cardiovascular activity before the examination. Temporal resolution is the key to a good scan (even more so than spatial resolution). Because the temporal resolution of CTA is limited at this time, the heart rhythm must be very slow and regular to optimize the scan. A preparation room to prepare the patient for intravenous (IV) placement and for IV β-blocker administration is useful if possible.

In patients with a pacemaker, it is helpful to set the lower rate limit to 60 bpm and β-block the patient to 100% paced, or to put a magnet on the chest, which will allow single-chamber (VVI) pacing (assuring a regular heart rate at the lower rate limit) and then scan the patient. Atrial and ventricular (AV) pacing should be attempted because AV dyssynchrony results in severe motion artifacts. In patients with long PR intervals, AV pacing with a shortened AV delay is preferred.

Metformin should be avoided (none for 24 hours before the scan) because of the potential adverse effects when used concomitantly with iodinated contrast agents. In addition, metformin should be held for 48 hours after contrast administration. Viagra, Cialis, and Levitra should also be avoided 48 hours before a CTA because nitrates are needed to dilate the coronary arteries. Premedication with Mucomyst is recommended if the creatinine is elevated (≥1.4). Finally, if a contrast allergy is present, premedication with steroids and antihistamines is required.

Be sure the electrocardiogram (ECG) leads are appropriately placed to avoid the typical ECG-lead imaging artifact and to assure an adequate ECG tracing. In addition, always confirm the function of the IV site (may be done at the time of the test bolus).

Patients must be relaxed (music, dimly lit room) for the scan. Anxiety is an issue and may add up to 15 beats per minute (bpm) to the initial resting heart rate. Therefore, β-block accordingly. Explain the procedure well and let the patient know what to expect. Warn them about the sensation during contrast injection. These steps will help reduce anxiety. The test bolus injection also helps because it may serve to prepare the patient for the full injection of contrast.

If the patient is particularly large, position him or her so the heart is in the center of the gantry where the X-ray beams are focused. In addition to increasing the mAs in large patients, turn off the dose-modulation function to increase the energy delivered to all phases of the cardiac cycle. By doing this, the number of phases available for analysis is increased.

Sublingual nitroglycerin, if not contraindicated, must be used to reduce the likelihood of poor visualization of the distal coronary arteries. This step is particularly crucial in patients with stents, in smokers, and in women and diabetics, both of which have inherently smaller coronary arteries. Prepare for the possibility that nitroglycerin may also increase the heart rate. The sublingual nitroglycerin (one or two tablets or sprays) should be administered just before the noncontrasted scan.

Finally, always perform a practice breath hold to identify heart rate changes during the breath hold that may occur during the final scan. Identification of any heart rate changes during the breath hold may permit further administration of β-blockers before the final CTA. The practice breath hold may be done during the noncontrasted scan.

Timing of the Scan

Scan timing in relation to the bolus injection is crucially important and depends on the clinical indication and the structure of interest. There are two ways to time the scan, the bolus tracking method and the test bolus method.

The bolus tracking method is performed by first placing a region of interest in the ascending or descending aorta. The onset of the final CTA scan is then set to begin when the contrast density (Hounsfield units) in the region of interest reaches a predefined threshold, usually 100–150 Hounsfield units. Disadvantages of this technique are that one has less control of the scan timing and the region of interest may accidently move to another inappropriate region such as the superior vena cava, throwing off the timing of the scan. A poorly timed scan will yield suboptimal contrast in the region of interest and thus make the scan nondiagnostic, whereas a properly timed scan will yield uniform contrast opacification and minimal artifacts. Finally, the bolus tracking technique does not allow a practice breath hold or a test of the IV site before the final contrast load. Remember, only one chance exists to obtain the images after contrast is injected.

The test bolus is our preferred method. It is performed by using 20 cc of contrast with a 25-cc flush at 5 cc/second, producing a small compact bolus. The preferred contrast injection sight is the right antecubital vein because the superior vena cava fills the heart from the right in most patients. Although the left antecubital vein can be used, the right-sided approach avoids contrast crossing over the anterior chest wall, which could interfere with analysis of the coronary arteries.

Low-dose sequential scans are then performed at the level of the ascending aorta (region of interest) at 2-second interscan intervals without overlap and the scan is terminated when the maximum intensity is reached. Usually, 10–15 snapshots are taken every 3/4 of a second. The initial scan delay after the test bolus contrast administration is about 7–10 seconds.

A contrast intensity curve is then formed and the timing of the scan is set based on the peak intensity of this curve (see Figure 6.2). The average time for the contrast to move from the injection site in the arm to the heart is approximately 15 seconds. If there is a severe decrease in a patient's cardiac output or if severe pulmonary hypertension exists, this delay has been as high as 50 seconds. The test bolus is necessary to gauge this time delay, which then drives the timing of the breath hold. The breath hold in general begins about 7 seconds after injection of contrast into the arm.

The general guidelines for appropriate scan timing are as follows (Figure 6.2). For imaging of the native coronary arteries, the scan is timed at +3 seconds after the contrast peak. If saphenous vein grafts are imaged, the timing is exactly at the peak (+0). The scan is started earlier than for the native coronaries because the scanned field of view (sFOV) is larger to include the ostia of the bypass grafts and thus the contrast must be imaged earlier. If a left internal mammary artery (LIMA) is imaged, the scan is timed to –1 second before the peak, because to image the origin of the LIMA, the sFOV must include the lung apices, so the scan must begin earlier to allow earlier visual-

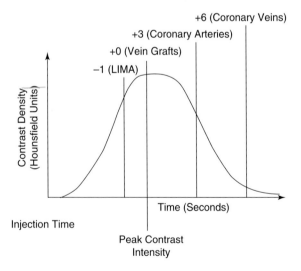

Figure 6.2. Timing of the cardiac CTA scan in relation to the peak contrast density of the test bolus for various structures of interest. The timing of the scan is crucial to successful cardiac CTA imaging.

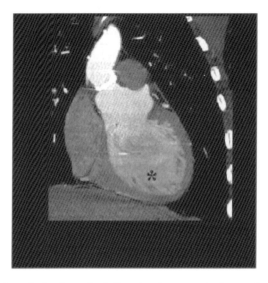

Figure 6.3. A poorly timed scan (late). Note that the contrast in the apex (asterisk) of the ventricle is less dense than in the aorta, which will result in poor opacification and thus poor visualization of the distal coronary arteries.

ization of contrast in this region. If the cardiac veins are imaged, the scan is then timed to +6 seconds after the peak to allow the contrast to pass through the coronary arteries and into the veins allowing their adequate visualization. These timing guidelines may be altered slightly if needed to optimize image quality.

Optimal scan timing will be apparent by noting a uniform, adequate (>350 Hounsfield units) contrast opacification throughout the entire ventricle and ascending aorta and is best assessed in the coronal plane. When interested in the coronary arteries, an inappropriate scan time delay (late imaging of the contrast) will permit the coronary veins to fill with contrast. The venous opacification and overlap with the coronary arteries will interfere with the visualization and assessment of the coronary arteries themselves. If the timing is too early, there is less contrast density in the ascending aorta than in the ventricle itself, resulting in poor opacification of the coronary arteries. If the timing is too late, there is less opacification in the apex of the heart than in the remaining part of the ventricle and aorta, resulting in poor visualization of the distal coronary arteries residing in these slabs. Figure 6.3 is an example of a poorly timed scan in which the scan was triggered to begin too late.

The three main factors that will degrade a CTA study are heart rate elevations and irregularity, incorrect contrast bolus and scan timing (crucial), and breathing or patient motion during the examination. The test bolus will allow optimization of all three variables before the final contrasted scan, thereby yielding the best chance for an optimal scan.

The Imaging Protocol

Prepare the patient in a holding room if possible. This will improve throughput efficiency. Take initial vital signs and place an 18-gauge IV in the right antecubital vein if possible. Administer per oral and/or IV β-blockers if needed. Place the patient on the scanner while explaining the procedure to the patient, including the sensation they may experience during contrast administration. Place the ECG leads in an optimal position to avoid artifact and to optimize the electrical tracing. Practice the breath hold while performing these tasks and while optimizing heart rate with further β-blockade if necessary. Lopressor at a dose of 5 mg every few minutes up to a maximum of 45–50 mg is reasonable. Most have found esmolol to be ineffective in this setting. Atenolol is also acceptable.

While preparing the patient for the scan, watch for heart rate variability and for arrhythmias. Nitroglycerin (1–2 doses) should be administered as a spray or sublingual tablet 5 minutes before the noncontrasted scan.

Next, obtain a CT topogram in one or two views (scout films). The topogram helps plan the sFOV. Some technologists prefer two scout views to help plan the sFOV. After the topogram, a noncontrasted scan is performed from the apex of the lungs to the adrenal glands, which may be reconstructed for radiology over read if needed. The usual requested reconstruction for the radiologist is in 3-mm slices, but can be reconstructed using thinner slices if needed. Evaluate the general calcium location and extent to determine if the contrasted scan will be useful. The next step is a bolus-timing curve or test bolus (usually 20 cc), which is used to time the final contrasted scan and may also be used for shunt analysis. Alternatively, the contrasted scan may be performed using the bolus tracking method. Finally, perform the contrasted scan.

Injection Techniques

There are multiple ways to perform the contrast bolus for the final CTA. The simplest method is a two-syringe dual injector technique in which syringe #1 is filled with contrast (enough for the test bolus and final contrast injection) and syringe #2 is filled with saline. After injecting the contrast syringe, the saline chaser is given (approximately 50 cc). The saline chaser is needed to keep the contrast moving continuously through the heart as a tight bolus.

Another method uses three syringes. The first syringe is filled with enough contrast to give the test bolus followed by the final contrast bolus. The second syringe is a mixture of contrast and saline and the third syringe is the final saline chaser. Specifically, the first syringe may be loaded with approximately 120 cc of contrast. After the 20-cc test bolus, the full contrast bolus volume is injected. Follow this injection by a mixture of 15 cc contrast and 35 cc of saline (total of 50 cc) as one injection at the same rate of the initial bolus injection. The third injection is the 50-cc saline chaser.

The injection rate for each injection is 5 cc/second most of the time. For small patients, the rate may be reduced to 4 cc/second and for large patients the rate is increased to 6–7 cc/second; 7 cc/second may only be used with an 18-gauge IV.

The injection volume is on average approximately 80 cc for the contrasted scan for average-size patients with creatinine values of <1.7 mg/dL. Volumes may be increased for larger patients (to increase the signal-to-noise ratio) and for patients with bypass grafts because the sFOV is larger. With a larger sFOV, the scan time will increase and thus the contrast volume will need to be increased (120 cc) in order to widen the bolus, which then ensures that contrast is present in the regions of interest throughout the entire scan. If the creatinine is ≥1.7, the contrast volume should be reduced to 60 cc.

The purpose of the triple syringe technique is to create mild contrast opacification of the right ventricle (to allow functional assessment of the right ventricle) without causing contamination of the coronary artery evaluation. The right ventricular contrast opacification should remain markedly less than that of the left ventricle. Also, this approach permits reasonable opacification of the pulmonary arteries to allow diagnosis of large pulmonary emboli.

Data Reconstruction

Data reconstruction is the process in which the technician converts the raw data into axial images. All data must first undergo a "cone beam" reconstruction to correct for the angular spread of the X-ray beams. In addition, the data undergo "back filtration and convolution" (see convolution filters below), which averages the scattered Gaussian data curves into data points. The operator may further select special reconstructions to enhance analysis such as multisegment reconstruction or multiphasic reconstruction (discussed below). The raw data can be revisited to provide other reconstructions if necessary. In other words, you get what you ask for from the data but you can go back for seconds if needed.

There are special problems that must be overcome by data reconstruction, which are enhanced by certain types of reconstruction algorithms. Discussed below are important problems to consider in CTA and their potential solutions. These discussions include problems with zoom, noise, motion, and variability.

Zoom Problems

Pixels that are spread out, made bigger, or duplicated will create zoom artifacts. Zoom artifacts distort the image and occur as the displayed FOV (dFOV) of the image is changed as discussed previously. One digital zoom is usually acceptable before image distortion and degradation occurs. After the first digital zoom, the image becomes blurry as artifact is introduced. The picture size is equivalent to the dFOV. In a 512×512 matrix, for example, there are a fixed number of voxels, namely 262,144 (512 squared). Because the heart size does not match the size of the screen, one can magnify the heart in a 1 : 1 manner to the size of the screen without compromise. Magnification without image compromise is accomplished by narrowing the scanned FOV (sFOV) to the size of the heart. This increases the number of pixels per centimeter of image improving the spatial resolution. This magnification is "free" so to speak, where each voxel represents one portion of the image. Digital zooming increases the number of voxels representing the same image portion, thus introducing distortion.

Noise Problems

The image quality in any imaging modality is directly related to the signal and inversely related to the amount of noise or scatter in the case of X-rays. Increased noise will make the image grainy. This will often be noticeable in obese patients. Increased noise will also be seen with poorer quality contrast or contrast with lower concentrations of iodine. Analyzing the image in the coronal view will allow for immediate analysis of the signal-to-noise ratio by paying particular attention to the graininess of the image. The coronal view also allows a determination of the evenness of the contrast throughout the heart and great vessels. Uneven contrast opacification (too little contrast or poorly timed contrast) will create problems. If the heart is imaged too early, the contrast will not have time to adequately opacify the distal coronary arteries and artifactual lesions (pseudo lesions) may be visualized. If the heart is imaged too late, too little contrast will be seen in the proximal coronary arteries (contrast has come and gone).

The solution to minimize noise (scatter) is the use of convolution filters. What follows below is a brief discussion of convolution filters. The voxel (three-dimensional pixel) is the smallest image display unit. Because of the inherent limitations and inaccuracy of X-ray detection (100% certainty concerning the origin of an X-ray beam cannot be obtained), the representation of the density of the attenuated X-ray by the voxel may be blurred. In other words, confidence in the validity of the information represented by an individual voxel is limited as evidenced by the fact that the density measurement within the voxel is not a perfect Gaussian curve.

To increase the confidence in the information within each voxel, density measurements from neighboring voxels are borrowed and added to the center voxel of interest to enhance the confidence in its density estimate. Therefore, each voxel's density measurement is actually a weighted average of itself and those voxels surrounding it (adding from its neighbors). By doing this, noise and scatter are reduced and the edges of the image are softened or blurred in the x and y axes. The compromise here is a reduced ability to see fine detail around the edges. The more weight given to neighboring voxels (more neighbors included in the center voxel estimate), the smoother or blurrier the image,

Matrix Size is 14 Voxels X 13 Voxels

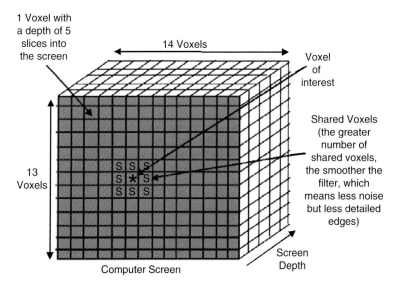

Figure 6.4. A cartoon depiction of filtering. Filtering kernels allow the sharing of neighboring voxels' information in calculating an estimate of the contrast density of the voxel of interest. The weight given to neighboring voxels determines the filter kernel type and characteristics.

resulting in less noise but the less fine detail around the edges as well (Figure 6.4).

There are three types of convolution filters. These filters work to improve the image in the x and y axes. The first is the normal kernel, which adds similar weight to the center voxel and the neighboring voxels. The second or soft kernel adds more significant weight to the neighbors, yielding a smoother, less noisy image while sacrificing fine detail at the edges. The last or sharp kernel adds less weight to the neighboring voxels. This is the noisiest filter, but yields better fine detail. This kernel works best for stents or for reading around bypass clips and significant calcium.

Slice thickening is another filtering method, which alternatively affects the z-axis rather than the x, y axes. In this case, increasing the number of slices viewed in a single image (thicker slices) will allow an averaging of data in the z-axis or through-plane (from top to bottom). The minimum slice thickness is approximately 0.6 mm. By thickening the slices, the noise is decreased in the through-plane with a concomitant blurring of the image in the same plane. In addition, slice thickening causes a loss of spatial resolution in the through-plane. This technique is known as maximal intensity projection (MIP) and is discussed below.

Therefore, if interested in the x- and y-plane (artery is running in this plane), the slice thickness may be increased to improve visualization. The blurring in the z-axis is less important because the point of interest is located in the x and y axes. If the point of interest is in the z-axis, smoother convolution filters may be used because the reader is less concerned about fine detail in the x-, y-plane.

Motion Problems

Motion makes the image blurry. Tachycardia, irregular heart rhythms, ectopy, failure to deal adequately with cardiac motion, and excessive patient motion or breathing during the scan will result in a blurred image with loss of fine detail. The goal is to, in essence, "freeze" the heart. The more success at this, the better the image will be.

There are many types of cardiac motion for which to correct. First, the patient must hold their breath during the scan. Breathing will alter the location of the chest wall and heart during the scan. Second, the heart itself moves in very complex ways during the cardiac cycle. Finally, the coronary arteries move significantly throughout the R-R interval. Motion during the cardiac cycle differs greatly among the three major coronary arteries (Figure 6.5).[24] The right coronary artery moves most significantly (average of 69.5 mm/second) followed by the circumflex (average of 48.4 mm/second) followed by the left anterior descending artery, which moves the least (average of 22.4 mm/second).[23] Even with cardiac catheterization, in which the temporal resolution is 8 ms, blurring of the right coronary artery still occurs. The best temporal resolution for a single-gantry rotation is approximately 87 ms [less for dual-source CT (DSCT)] which enhances motion artifact.

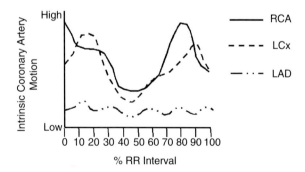

Figure 6.5. Graph of coronary motion throughout the cardiac cycle. The right coronary artery (RCA) demonstrates the most intrinsic motion. LCx, left circumflex artery; LAD, left anterior descending coronary artery.

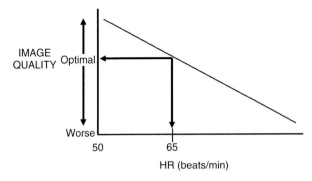

Figure 6.6. Graphic depiction of heart rate (HR) as it relates to image quality. The optimal heart rate for cardiac CTA imaging is near 65 bpm.

There are two ways to help deal with cardiac motion: Slow the heart rate down or alter the reconstruction method. The best technique is to slow down the heart rate. β-blockers are excellent for this purpose. Calcium channel blockers are acceptable in the rare patient who has a contraindication to β-blockers. In general, atenolol and metoprolol are the best β-blockers for this purpose but esmolol is ineffective in this application. In addition to improving image quality, β-blockers also reduce radiation exposure by allowing the use of dose modulation.

At this time, the optimal heart rate for cardiac CTA is 65 bpm and will likely not change with DSCT or increased numbers of detector rows (256-slice CT scanners). Despite adequate heart rate control, cardiac motion remains a difficult problem because there are many uncontrollable contributing factors such as the force of cardiac motion (dP/dT). The dP/dT of the moving heart may be high despite a slow heart rate, resulting in image degradation in the presence of adequate β-blockade.

The heart rate can also be too slow. Severe bradycardia (≤50 bpm) should be avoided. If the heart rate is <50 bpm, the pitch may need to be reduced if possible so as not to outrun the contrast bolus. A heart rate of 50–65 bpm is probably the "sweet spot" (Figure 6.6). Be aware that the heart rate will increase with the infusion of contrast, with IV placement, and with patient anxiety. Therefore, if the resting heart rate is 65 or greater, more β-blockers will be necessary to blunt this response.

If heart rate reduction is unsuccessful or incomplete, the technologist may use various reconstruction techniques to help deal with heart rate problems. These are described below.

Half Scan Integral Reconstruction

This technique is always used. By using half-gantry rotation (180-degree projections around the gantry), the time necessary to obtain an image is reduced to 155–160 ms, thus improving the temporal resolution of the scan.

Multisegment Reconstruction

In cardiac CTA, as discussed above, the goal is to scan the heart at the quietest time in the cardiac cycle. Generally, half-gantry rotation (with single-source CT scanners) occurs during each heartbeat. If instead, two consecutive beats are used to create a full half-gantry rotation (quarter-gantry rotation per heart beat), the temporal resolution is reduced to 87.5 ms. However, this method requires twice the time to scan the heart and thus exposes the patient to twice the radiation. Multisegment reconstruction can, in fact, be performed using up to 4 beats (1/8-gantry rotation per beat), improving the effective temporal resolution to 65 ms. This technique is still almost 10 times slower than cardiac catheterization.

For multisegmental reconstruction to be successful, the R-R interval must be very steady. If there is beat-to-beat variability, the image will still be blurred. Because images from two separate beats are required for multisegment reconstruction to complete one image slab, these two images must occur at exactly the same time within the cardiac cycle for each beat. If there is heart rate variability for any reason, the two separate images needed for the single slab will occur at separate points in the cardiac cycle, causing blurring of the image after reconstruction (Figures 6.7 and 6.8).

Unfortunately, with single-source CT scanners, multisegment reconstruction achieves an improved temporal resolution only at certain heart rates: 66,

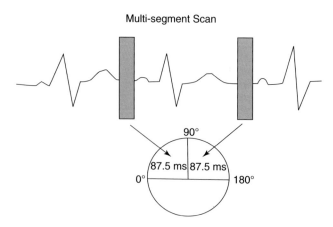

Figure 6.7. Multisegment reconstruction in which a quarter-gantry rotation occurs with each heart beat, and therefore, two heart beats are required to complete half of a gantry rotation (necessary for 360-degree cardiac imaging). This reconstruction technique effectively improves temporal resolution but requires a perfectly regular heart rhythm.

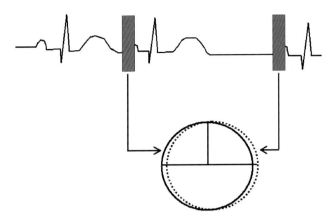

Figure 6.8. The effect of an irregular heart rhythm when using multisegment reconstruction. An irregular rhythm will result in blurring of the image because different cardiac cycles will be imaged during the two successive beats required for a half-gantry rotation.

81, and 104 bpm for a gantry rotation of 330 ms. For DSCT, multisegment reconstruction proves beneficial for many more heart rates, thus demonstrating an increased usefulness in a broader range of heart rates (Figure 6.9).[19]

Current CT scanners allow retrospective use of multisegment reconstruction techniques. There are no good data on the accuracy of multisegmental reconstruction scans.

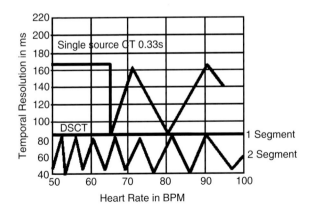

Figure 6.9. The limited utility of multisegment reconstruction when using a single-source CT scanner in which only selective heart beats permit the use of this reconstruction technique. With dual-source CT scanners, multisegment reconstruction is permitted with a wider range of heart rates. (Reprinted from Flohr et al.,[19] © 2006 Elsevier Ireland Ltd., with permission.)

Multiphasic Analysis

Another essential method to deal with cardiac motion is to use a multiphasic approach to image interpretation. Most cardiac motion occurs during systole. The least motion occurs during the preatrial kick at end-diastole. Therefore, the raw data can be reconstructed at various points or phases within the cardiac cycle to find the quietest times (i.e., at 10%, 20%, 30%, etc. of the cardiac cycle). Callister et al. have determined that in the majority of cases, the best phases for image interpretation are either 70% and 75% or 40% and 48% (Callister, The Tennessee Heart and Vascular Institute, unpublished oral communication, November 4, 2005). There may be different quiet times for different coronary arteries. Sometimes the right coronary artery is best visualized in end-systole (approximately 40%) whereas the left anterior descending artery may be best seen at end-diastole (approximately 70%). These generalizations sometimes do not apply and the left anterior descending artery is best seen closer to systole and vice versa for the right coronary artery.

Multiphasic reconstruction is also used to evaluate ejection fraction in which multiple phases from end-diastole to end-systole are analyzed to assess the global and regional function of the heart.

Some physicians routinely analyze 20 cardiac phases from 0% to 95% in 5% intervals (Figure 6.10) (M. Poon, Cabrini Medical Center, New York, NY, unpublished oral communication, February 6, 2006). The more reconstructed phases, however, the more time it takes to load them to the workstation, and more space is required to save the data. The hardware and workstation software must be powerful enough to handle all of the data. In addition, this type of analysis requires an adequate storage system to handle this massive amount of information.

Callister will usually reconstruct at 0%, 40%, 48%, 73%, and 78%. In 1 of 20 scans, he will need to go back to the technician to reconstruct other phases (Callister, The Tennessee Heart and Vascular Institute, unpublished oral communication, November 1, 2005). Others advocate that if a phase is determined

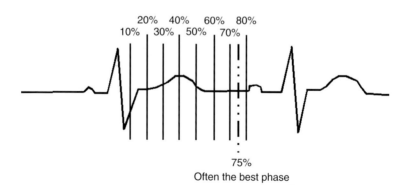

Figure 6.10. Various imaging phases within the cardiac cycle and clarification of the concept of percent of the R-R interval.

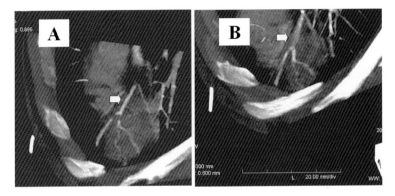

Figure 6.11. The LAD imaged during two separate cardiac phases in the same patient. **A** The proximal LAD (white arrow) is clearly visualized. **B** The LAD is blurred because of motion (white arrow). LAD, left anterior descending artery.

to be adequate to eliminate motion artifact in the mid right coronary artery (the mid right coronary artery typically demonstrates the most motion), then that par-ticular phase will likely be adequate for the analysis of all the coronary arteries (Budoff, UCLA Medical Center, Los Angeles, CA, unpublished oral communication, May 1, 2006).

We have found that using multiphasic reconstruction is best, in which 20 phases are routinely reconstructed at 5% intervals from 0% to 95% and loaded onto the workstation simultaneously. This provides the ability to easily click through different phases when needed. Poon suggests that often you will need different phases are needed to best see different parts of even the same coronary artery because of motion artifact, which varies even within the same coronary artery (Figure 6.11) (M. Poon, Cabrini Medical Center, New York, NY, unpublished oral communication, February 1, 2006). For practical purposes, 20 phases at 5% intervals is the best that can be presently done and this approach tends to be more than adequate. Note that there may be phasic differences with as little as a 2% phase shift.

Also be aware that at times, to read around artifacts, it is necessary to evaluate each image slab separately using different phases and different reconstruction techniques and filters.

Variability Problems

Variability problems include excess heart rate variability, cardiac arrhythmias, patient motion or breathing motion, or poor ECG adjustment. Because the entire heart is not scanned at the same time but rather in segments, the heart must be at the same point in the cardiac cycle each time a different segment is scanned. In addition, the heart must also be in the same location

HR after maximum B Blocker

		<70	>70
HR variablity of >10 beats with breath hold	Yes	Single Segment Scan	Multi-segment scan
	No	Single segment scan and use lidocaine (50 mg for a small patient and 100 mg for a large patient right before the scan) if PVCs are present. If significant heart rate variability issues, use atropine (0.7 mg if mild or 1 mg if severe). These measures work 75% of the time.	No win situation. Multi-segment scan will worsen image. HR will be too fast for single segment scan. Therefore, use both reconstruction methods and do the best you can to find the best phases for each difficult segment of artery.

Figure 6.12. An algorithm for dealing with various heart rates and heart rate variabilities when attempting to acquire a cardiac CTA image. PVC, premature ventricular contraction.

within the chest cavity during the scanning of each segment, which may be affected by breathing motion. If these criteria are not adequately met, there will be problems with reconstructing the various scanned segments to create a truthful image of the entire heart.

Problems with variability will create streak artifacts or misregistration artifacts. Once this occurs, there is not much that can be done after the fact to correct the problem. One must do their best to read around and through these problematic artifacts. Figure 6.12 depicts an algorithm for correcting potential imaging problems.

Image Display

The last step in the creation of a cardiac CTA image is the image display, which involves reformatting the images at the workstation to allow interpretation, and is generally performed by the physician. Each physician develops his or her own style or series of display orientations. Display orientations include the viewing angle and display format from which you look at the image. Options include three-dimensional multiplanar reconstruction, also known as volume rendering technique (VRT), and various two-dimensional analysis formats, including multiplanar reformatting (MPR), maximal intensity projections (MIPs), oblique MPR, and curved MPR. These reconstruction options are discussed in detail below. Keep in mind that reconstructions are useful, but potentially hazardous, thus their limitations must always be kept in mind during image interpretation.

Three-Dimensional Multiplanar Reconstruction (Volume Rendering)

VRT is a three-dimensional display format in which all voxels greater than a predetermined Hounsfield unit level will be displayed and each of these voxels is assigned an intensity value for opacity based on its CT density (Figure 6.13). Subsequently, each intensity value is assigned a gray scale value or is color coded, and displayed in two dimensions. This technique uses lighting effects to shade and color the surface structures to create a three-dimensional depiction. Increased intensity voxels are more opaque and less intense voxels are more translucent.

VRT allows the reader to step back and visualize the gross anatomy of surface structures only. Think of the VRT format as looking at the forest through the trees. It helps for orientation purposes and to obtain general anatomic information. It may also be used to check for artifacts in order to quickly assess the best phase for analysis. VRT should not be used in isolation to make a diagnosis per se. This technique is not very sensitive for displaying stenoses but it is quite specific. If a lesion is apparent in the VRT image, and an artifact cannot explain the finding, the lesion is usually real. Positive remodelling always indicates the presence of underlying atheroma.

The newest software packages use "isotropic voxels" in which the collimation is the same in all dimensions ($0.6 \times 0.6 \times 0.6$ mm). By using isotropic voxels, the same resolution is present in any plane and in any orientation, thus allowing free rotation of the image without distortion.

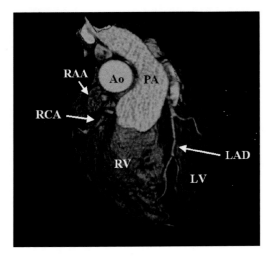

Figure 6.13. A good example of a VRT image. Note the left ventricle (LV), the right ventricle (RV), the right atrial appendage (RAA), the aorta (Ao), the pulmonary artery (PA), the left anterior descending artery (LAD), and the right coronary artery (RCA).

Maximum Intensity Projection

This is another display type, which may be thought of as coning down to look at the individual trees and not the whole forest. MIP uses voxels that are multiple slices thick, which are called slabs (Figures 6.14 and 6.15). These slabs project deep into the screen. The brightest voxel in the slab is automatically selected and moved to the front of the slab to be viewed on the screen. In other words, all the gray scale density information is contained in the image but the brightest density in each voxel from any of the slices is brought forward to the screen and is the only density visualized (the original density data remain within the image without fancy manipulations). The thickness of the MIP (slab thickness) is determined by the user and mandates the number of slices in the slab (because each slice has a predetermined thickness). Any imaging angle may be chosen so the image may be freely rotated. MIP is essentially a three-dimensional MPR several slices thick.

MIP is a great way to navigate through the course of the coronary arteries, and therefore it allows a general overview of the coronary artery anatomy so that potential problem areas in need of further analysis may be identified (using MPR). By bringing the brightest contrast to the forefront, the lumen will appear as large and as bright as it can possibly be. Therefore, if a tight

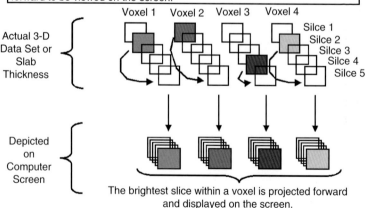

Figure 6.14. Cartoon depiction of the MIP reconstruction format.

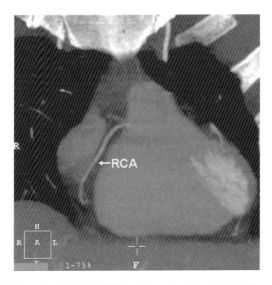

Figure 6.15. Illustration of a thin MIP (6 mm) reconstruction of the right coronary artery (RCA). Note the similarity to an angiographic appearance.

stenosis is seen in MIP display (without artifact), the lesion is truly severe. Thus, MIP is specific for tight lesions but not sensitive, as stenoses can be missed because multiple slices are combined, thereby potentially hiding subtle abnormalities.

The slab thickness used for navigation through the coronary arteries is a personal preference issue and may be varied. In fact, one may use different slab thickness while deciphering different areas in the same coronary artery. Regions with overlap (i.e., the proximal circumflex is often hidden by the left atrial appendage) will require thinner MIP analysis to adequately visualize. Callister uses an MIP slab thickness of approximately 5 mm, which causes less overlap of structures but makes navigation slightly more cumbersome (Callister, The Tennessee Heart and Vascular Institute, unpublished oral communication, November 4, 2005). Poon uses an MIP of 15, which allows easy navigation but may require thinner MIP thicknesses for areas of overlap (M. Poon, Cabrini Medical Center, New York, NY, unpublished oral communication, February 6, 2006). The thicker the MIP used, the more practical image navigation becomes at the expense of reduced sensitivity.

To prevent overlooking soft plaque or subtle abnormalities, focus in on the lumen edge. If the lumen edge is smooth with no evidence of positive or negative remodeling, then there is a very low likelihood of soft plaque. Always look in two oblique views as is done with cardiac catheterization projections.

Single-Plane Multiplanar Reconstruction

MPR allows narrowing in further on the image as if one were looking at the individual leaves of a single tree. The image format represents a single-voxel-thick straight line through the image. It displays all the voxels in a given chosen plane one slice at a time. VRT is the most general overview. MIP is a little more focused. MPR is the most focused, providing the most detail, but the MPR format is difficult for general navigation because one can easily lose perspective.

MPR represents the actual raw data and is used to focus in and make a diagnosis. The axial MPR images are not prone to misregistration. Although MPR is best for looking at fine detail and for making diagnoses, one can easily get lost in the image because the reader is confined to looking at a very thin slice. One cannot start from an MPR image because interpretation would be tantamount to finding a needle in a haystack. Therefore, the VRT and the MIP reconstructions are used to give orientation and to guide the reader to spots of particular interest (potential problem areas). MPR is then used to focus in and make a diagnosis, thus confirming the general findings of MIP and VRT. MPR yields better resolution of soft plaque edges at the expense of a potential increase in noise. Be sure to rotate around the entire vessel in MPR using multiple views and scrolling through multiple image slices. A prudent professional will not rely on MIP alone.

MPR is the gold standard for making a diagnosis but VRT and MIP reconstruction techniques are essential because if problem areas cannot be found, they cannot be diagnosed.

Oblique Multiplanar Reconstruction

To visualize very small objects such as coronary arteries, rotation through many imaging planes is necessary. In fact, in order to remain oriented while viewing the images, one needs to rotate around an actual center point (center point of rotation), and not simply rotate the whole plane itself. Current workstations allow the operator to choose any straight oblique viewing plane through the three-dimensional image dataset with a subsequent single slice display in the chosen imaging plane. Oblique MPR allows the reader to navigate through the data in any plane (rotate the image), which is necessary to follow anatomic structures through the dataset (for example, coronary arteries, which do not remain in standard imaging planes) (Figure 6.16).

In oblique MPR the reader angles through the original, axial dataset in any straight angle creating a single slice image along the chosen viewing plane. This plane may be freely rotated, allowing real-time navigation along the course of a coronary artery. Oblique MPR may also be performed using thicker slices, tantamount to an MIP, to simplify navigation. This type of display demands a powerful workstation to allow movement of the image concomitantly with movement of the mouse without delay. If the workstation images lag behind the mouse movement, the software is not powerful enough and

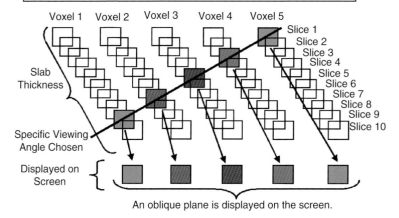

Figure 6.16. Cartoon depiction of the oblique MPR reconstruction format.

analysis will be difficult. Oblique MPR allows intuitive interpretation of cardiac CTA images.

Curved Multiplanar Reconstruction

Curved MPR displays a single-pixel-thick curved line through a specifically chosen course through the image (such as through the course of a coronary artery), creating a straight-line reformation of the entire vessel from origin to termination, and simultaneously displaying the image in two orthogonal projections (Figures 6.17 and 6.18). This technique artificially straightens a curved structure and displays it on the screen as a straight line. The reader must be permitted to freely rotate around the straightened image to avoid artifacts and pitfalls. Curved MPR is the display format used for tree renderings and vessel tracing techniques.

This display format can, however, distort the image. It may disorient the reader, causing a loss of anatomic context. In addition, curved MPR can also create the appearance of artifacts (pseudo lesions) by hiding tortuosity and branching points, for example. In other words, the end product of this display reconstruction is wholly dependent on the computer's ability to correctly follow a chosen course through the dataset and display it correctly. This reconstruction involves a significant amount of data manipulation. This display format works best with isotropic voxels.

In this cartoon, each voxel depicted on the computer screen is 10 slices thick. If the screen is a 512 by 512 matrix, there would be 512 voxels across the screen and 512 voxels down the screen. The curved MPR format projects a single, user defined, line through the image in any number of chosen planes and displays this curved line onto the computer screen as a single plane of voxel densities. Since this is an MPR format, the resulting image is one plane thick.

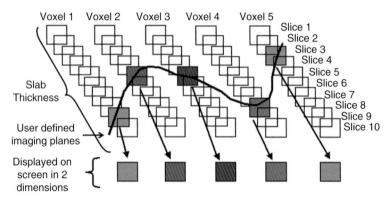

Figure 6.17. Cartoon depiction of the curved MPR reconstruction format.

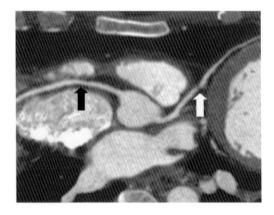

Figure 6.18. A curved MPR representation of the right coronary artery (black arrow) and left coronary artery (white arrow). Note that the artery is artificially straightened and displayed in two dimensions on one screen. Incidentally, the LAD may have a tight stenosis. This representation alone would be insufficient to confirm a tight lesion.

Some experts believe that curved MPR is not useful at all. Others use the technique when needed, while recognizing its limitations and difficulties. With certain workstations, curved MPR may be very time consuming.

Black and White Reversal

The color scheme of the display may be reversed where bright objects are displayed as black and vice versa. This technique may be helpful in special circumstances such as valve motion analysis.

Four-Dimensional Analysis (Multiphasic Analysis)

With this technique all cardiac phases are loaded into the analysis software package workstation. With this technique, nearly 6000 images are loaded in 20 phases at 5% intervals from 0% to 95% at every 5% with approximately 300 pictures in each phase.

The best phase for general analysis is selected based on the characteristics determined by VRT or MIP displays, in which the phase with the least motion and the least number of artifacts is selected. One can play all the phases in a cine loop to quickly establish the optimal phase. When a stenosis is suspected, it can be viewed quickly in all phases to exclude artifact and motion as the cause of the finding. The reader simply clicks through all of the phases, one at a time. It is not uncommon that the reader will need to evaluate the coronary arteries in a piecemeal manner in which different parts of the artery are examined in different phases.

At this time, the multiphasic analysis works best with the TeraRecon workstation. In time, other workstations will become more robust and will likely allow this type of analysis. This analysis technique does not preclude the need for adequate heart rate control and for meticulous attention to detail in the patient preparation and scan acquisition. It should also be noted that others, such as Budoff, have not adopted this technique as necessary, citing that the phase with the least motion in the mid right coronary artery will likely be an adequate phase for complete analysis of all the coronary arteries (Budoff, UCLA Medical Center, Los Angeles, CA, unpublished oral communication, May 1, 2006).

The newest Toshiba CT scanners are capable of automatically selecting the optimal phase (least motion) for each coronary artery. Only these phases need to be transferred to the work station. This propietary feature is called Phase Xact.

Virtual Angioscopy

This tool provides a virtual intraluminal tour (Figure 6.19).

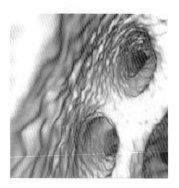 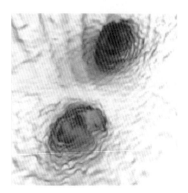

Figure 6.19. The vessel view format, which essentially is an intracavitary or intravessel view.

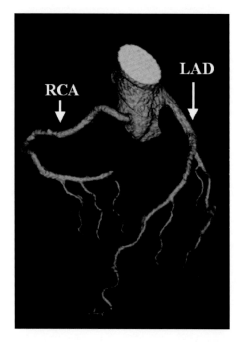

Figure 6.20. The typical vessel tree created by autosegmentation. The heart itself is absent from the image. This image is depicted in the VRT mode. It may also be viewed in MIP or MPR.

Tomographic Intravascular Analysis

Tomographic intravascular analysis (TIVA) is an experimental CTA technique in which Hounsfield units are used to determine plaque morphology. This technique is not yet ready for prime time but CTA has the potential for this analysis, pending further study. Thus, cardiac CTA may give a better sense of the complexity of an atherosclerotic lesion.

There is a good correlation between TIVA and IVUS (with IVUS, a lumen area of ≤6 mm indicates a critical stenosis). At times, the invasive angiogram may be wrong and the true nature of the stenosis is best seen by IVUS or CTA. Eventually, characterization of the plaque will aid in interventional planning because it may provide a foreshadowing of what the interventionalist must deal with during the procedure. Once again, TIVA is at this time experimental.

Autosegmentation

All information is removed from the image except the arteries. A vessel tree is created without the remaining cardiac image (Figure 6.20). The vessel tree may then be viewed in a VRT, MIP, or MPR format (with selected workstations such as General Electric). The vessel tree may also be used for quick navigation through the coronary arteries to identify potential problem areas that need further analysis. Budoff tends to use this approach (Budoff, UCLA Medical Center, Los Angeles, CA, unpublished oral communication, May 1, 2006).

7. A Systematic Approach to Reading and Reporting a Cardiac CTA Scan

It is essential to develop a systematic approach to reading cardiac computed tomographic angiography (CTA) scans, or important findings will surely be missed. Each reader may develop his or her own personal reading style. Suggested below is one possible systematic approach to reading a cardiac CTA scan.

Scan Quality

Discuss quality of the scan. Ask the questions "Is the scan useful and can it be relied on?" and "What are the limitations of this particular scan?" These questions can be easily answered by going to the volume rendering technique (VRT) reconstruction and quickly looking at the chest wall for motion artifacts caused by breathing, which will be most evident as step artifacts or misregistration. Next, slice through the chest to the heart in the VRT mode and look for cardiac motion artifacts or arrhythmia artifacts, evident as misregistration seen on the heart itself. If multiple phases are loaded, the reader may also play a loop through all of the phases in the VRT format to get a quick idea of the integrity of the data in different phases. In addition, a rapid analysis of the quality of the image in the region of the distal arteries can be performed. Look at the axial data in multiplanar reformatting (MPR) or maximal intensity projection (MIP) to assess for "jumps" in the data. If present, the data in the slices bordering the "jumps" may be flawed and particular care must be taken when assessing these regions.

Then look at the coronal slices in thin MIP. This will help with assessment of the adequacy and evenness of the contrast enhancement and with the timing of the scan. By doing this, problems with image interpretation in certain scan regions may be anticipated. The contrast density in the ascending aorta and throughout the left ventricle should be ≥350 Hounsfield units and should be uniform and even. If the Hounsfield units are markedly <350 in the ascending aorta and ventricle, the contrast enhancement may be inadequate to allow diagnostic imaging of the coronary arteries. If there is too little contrast in the apex of the left ventricle, then the timing was late. In this case, marked coronary venous contamination will occur. Furthermore, the coronary artery contrast opacification may be suboptimal. If there is too little contrast in the ascending aorta, then the timing was too early and the coronary arteries may be inadequately opacified. This may cause the appearance of pseudo-lesions.

In the coronal thin MIP, the noise level may be assessed as well. Assess for graininess in the image, representing noise or scatter. If the image is grainy, the fix would have been to increase the mAs to give more radiation, thus improving the signal-to-noise ratio. Increase the mAs prospectively in large patients.

The coronal orientation is also a good place to check for cardiac motion or image blurriness. Immediately look at the mid right coronary artery, which demonstrates the most motion. If this artery looks round and anatomically correct, chances are that this particular phase will be the most optimal one in general. The technologist may be trained to automatically perform this assessment and provide the reader with the best phase. If a suboptimal phase is identified, moving backward toward end-systole by 5% phase increments (minimum phase of about 40%) will ultimately yield the best phase. As the heart rate increases, phases closer to end-systole will be required.

The fix for increased cardiac motion would be to give more β-blockers to assure a heart rate of ≤65 bpm during the scan. The scan may potentially be rescued by reconstructing in the multisegment reconstruction format. Alternatively, the reader must hunt for different reconstruction phases that allow better visualization of various regions of interest. Different coronary segments may be optimally seen in different cardiac phases. Softer filters may also be used to help overcome limitations but the trade-offs previously discussed must be considered.

Finally, look for variability artifacts, which also appear as misregistration. The fix for variability problems is also to administer more β-blocker. In addition, lidocaine may be given for premature ventricular contractions. Atropine often helps for sinus arrhythmia. Proper electrocardiogram (ECG) lead placement is also required. Unfortunately, there is not a good rescue for variability problems. Readers may need to evaluate each image slice between reconstruction seams independently using different phases and varying reconstruction techniques. This process may be very time-consuming. The lesson here is that adequate time spent preparing the patient before the scan will most certainly pay off in the end.

Coronary Artery and Bypass Graft Analysis

The next step is to analyze the coronary arteries and bypass grafts if present. In the axial plane, the right coronary artery arises at 10 o'clock or closer to noon if there is an anterior take-off. The left main coronary artery arises at 3 o'clock. The left anterior descending originates at 2 o'clock and the circumflex at 5 o'clock. Dominance may also be established in the axial plane. Finally, the axial plane will help identify the conus artery, which originates from the proximal right coronary artery and moves upward versus an atrial branch, which also originates from the proximal right coronary artery but moves downward.

Analysis of the coronary arteries may be easier and less time-consuming by starting with templates to optimize the initial image orientation when beginning to assess each artery and graft (if present). Templates are easily created with the TeraRecon workstation by using an MIP overlay on the VRT (an existing function) to find a desired three-dimensional orientation. Next, switch to MPR or MIP and save the template. Other companies will follow with workstations that are as powerful as the TeraRecon. The prudent reader will save significant time by creating templates for all structures to be read in the normal reading workflow.

Use the calcium score (CaSc) to help evaluate the coronaries. If the CaSc is 0, only 1 in 1000 patients will have a tight stenosis unless the patient is ≤40 years of age when all bets are off (Budoff, UCLA Medical Center, Los Angeles, CA, unpublished oral communication, May 1, 2006). Therefore, the CaSc may shift the pretest probability of finding a significant coronary lesion. Thus, for practical purposes, if debating between lesions versus artifact, the CaSc may sway the decision. It should be noted that a CaSc of 0 does not guarantee no atherosclerosis or the absence of a flow-limiting stenosis.

Utilize MIP (thick or thin) to navigate the coronary arteries and bypass grafts. Attempt to lay them out in orientations similar to cardiac angiography. Cardiac CTA must live up to the gold standard of cardiac catheterization, and standard angiographic orientations applied to CTA will make interpretation of the CTA much simpler and more plausible. MIP reconstructions are great for in-plane arteries but if looking at an artery in cross-section, the MIP is useless because an arterial short axis in MIP represents a column of dye, thereby rendering it impossible to diagnose a focal lesion. An artery in cross-section requires MPR reconstructions to diagnose lesions because each MPR image represents one single image slice.

When navigating the arterial tree in thick MIP, look for irregularities in the artery or for positive or negative remodeling to provide clues to potential problem areas. The thicker the MIP, the greater likelihood that subtle areas of soft plaque will be overlooked. Major stenoses, however, will usually be associated with either positive or negative remodeling. We have found that an MIP of 5–7 mm is best for a general navigational overview. Other readers will use an MIP of 15 mm (M. Poon, Cabrini Medical Center, New York, NY, unpublished oral communication, February 6, 2006). Some experts will first scan the arteries in the vessel tree mode to identify areas of concern, utilizing the same concepts (Budoff, UCLA Medical Center, Los Angeles, CA, unpublished oral communication, May 1, 2006). Still others will simply scan the arteries in the axial plane using MPR to identify problem areas, switching to other imaging planes and reconstruction formats if problem areas arise (D. Ropers, Department of Cardiology, University of Erlangen-Nurnberg, unpublished oral communication, April 6, 2006).

For practical purposes, one must develop a personal method of quickly navigating through the coronary tree to identify problem areas that need more analysis. If an artery has smooth contours and no potential problems are identified, feel comfortable moving on to the next artery because the likelihood of significant disease in this artery is low. The practical reality is that time is limited and it is not reasonable to spend significant time on areas that have a low likelihood of significant atherosclerosis. Maximize efficiency by giving particular attention only to areas of concern. In addition, once an area that mandates angiography is found, limit the time spent on the remainder of the arterial tree because a clinical decision has already been made.

Once problem areas are identified, use the thinner MIP and finally MPR to narrow down on the problem and confirm a diagnosis. Be sure to rule out artifacts. Remember, abnormalities should be assumed to be artifactual until proven otherwise. With MPR, always scroll through all the slices that make up the arterial thickness so that very focal stenoses will be identified. For example, if the artery is 3 mm and one is using MPR, the minimum slice thickness is approximately 0.4–0.6 mm. Therefore, there will be at least five slices that make up the entire arterial thickness. Scrolling through all of the slices will minimize the chance for error. If dye is seen in only one or two of the five slices, the lesion must be tight.

Curved MPR techniques may also be useful to confirm abnormalities but keep in mind its hazards and limitations. In the catheterization laboratory, the tightest view is the right answer. Because CTA is a tomographic technique and not a projection, here, the view that provides the maximum lumen is the correct answer.

Be sure to look at the entire artery in two orthogonal planes as is done in the catheterization laboratory (Figure 7.1). In general, any area of interest should be converted to a short-axis view of the artery before making a final diagnosis (Figure 7.2). Also, any abnormality should be confirmed in all phases before making a diagnosis. If only limited phases for analysis are available, make a disclaimer to this effect in your read. Also, vessels that are <1.5 mm

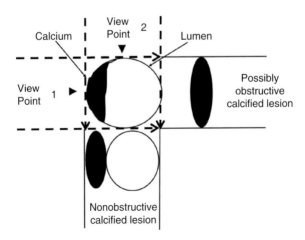

Figure 7.1. Demonstration of the need for two orthogonal views when analyzing a coronary lesion. Plaques and or calcium may be eccentric and the percent stenosis may vary depending on the viewing plane. In this example, the artery appears occluded in viewpoint 1 but proves nonobstructive in viewpoint 2.

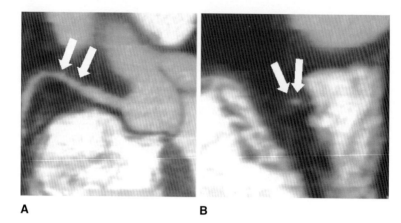

A   **B**

Figure 7.2. Soft plaque in a coronary artery (yellow arrows) in long axis **(A)** and short axis **(B)**. A short-axis view should always be performed to confirm an abnormal finding.

or so are not accurately assessed so do not waste time on arteries of this size. Only analyze an artery as far out distally as possible. Do not comment (or provide a disclaimer) on segments that are inadequately visualized. Cardiac catheterization will visualize more distal segments of a coronary artery than what is possible with CTA.

Sometimes the left main coronary artery is difficult to adequately analyze. The left main is best viewed from the top down. A view like this may be obtained by starting with the VRT images. Rotate the heart so that it is viewed from above and then cut through the heart until the left main is visualized. Often the proximal circumflex is hidden by the overlapping left atrial appendage. Thinner MIP techniques will eliminate this overlap and allow adequate analysis of this segment.

At times, the distal coronary arteries will be poorly seen. If so, the potential reasons include small distal arteries (diffuse disease, diabetics, smokers, and women), failure to administer nitroglycerin tight proximal lesions, too little contrast, a poorly timed scan, motion, or a suboptimal phase.

Cardiac Structure

First analyze the four-chamber view. In this view, cardiac chamber size and myocardial thickness may be assessed. In addition, right ventricular myocardium may be analyzed. Fatty infiltration and scarring can be seen. Shunts such as atrial septal defects may also be identified. Prominent right heart borders may be seen and can be caused by right atrial diverticula, which are normal variants.

Analyze the pericardium. It should be <4 mm thick. A mildly thickened pericardium isolated to the area around the right atrium is a normal finding. Rule out a pericardial effusion. Transudate cannot be reliably differentiated from exudate by Hounsfield unit measurement. However, blood will be approximately +30 Hounsfield units and serum or water density is close to 0 Hounsfield units.

Next, move to a short-axis template at the level of the aortic valve. Assess the structure of the aortic valve including the number of leaflets. By moving through various cardiac phases, leaflet movement can be assessed and aortic stenosis can be identified. Planimetry may be performed. Comment on aortic valve calcium.

Now look at the three-chamber view to evaluate the left ventricular outflow tract to rule out systolic anterior motion of the mitral valve. Follow this with the two-chamber template to look at the mitral valve and identify mitral annular calcification if present. The mitral valve can also be set in motion to see mitral valve thickening and even mitral valve prolapse. The mitral valve may also be assessed in short axis. Next, evaluate the left atrial appendage and pulmonary veins. With the TeraRecon workstation, an MIP-VRT overlay will easily orient the reader to these structures.

Finally, review the axial data to evaluate the ascending and descending aorta and the pulmonary artery at the level of the bifurcation. Comment on calcification, dilation (aneurysms), and dissections. All three great arteries should be roughly the same size. Look for the "bad boy" or any great artery that may be different from the others. The ascending aorta is the most common aberrancy. It is acceptable for the ascending aorta to be up to 1.3 times the size of the descending aorta after age 50. Be sure to assess the entire aorta. For example, if the descending aorta is very small, rule out coarctation. Rib notching and collateral chest vessels may be visualized. Suspect pulmonary hypertension if the pulmonary arteries are enlarged.

Remember that contiguous structures are attached. If the anatomy becomes confusing and orientation is lost, following a structure upward or downward to identify its origin and the other structures to which it attaches will frequently help to clarify anatomy.

Perfusion

Cardiac CTA is a reasonable noninvasive technique to detect myocardial infarction and should be part of the routine CTA analysis. In fact, cardiac CTA has been demonstrated to detect acute infarction with good accuracy.[25] It is superior to positron emission tomography (PET) and to single photon emission computed tomography (SPECT) because the resolution of CT is better than that of PET (7 mm) or SPECT (7–14 mm). With magnetic resonance imaging (MRI), delayed hyperenhancement of the myocardium with gadolinium appears white. With PET scanning, wall thinning correlates with lack of viability and if the wall thickness is ≤5 mm, there is near 0% chance for viability. Decreased perfusion of the myocardium with CTA appears dark and

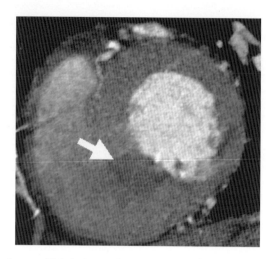

Figure 7.3. An area of inferior hypoperfusion or infarction (white arrow). Note the diminished contrast intensity in the inferior wall compared with the remainder of the myocardium.

represents first-pass hypoenhancement (Figure 7.3). First-pass enhancement of the myocardium with CTA normally appears relatively bright. To accomplish perfusion analysis, use MPR because very thin slices are required. In addition, only perform this analysis in the axial dataset.

The Hounsfield unit level of normal myocardium is near 100. The septum is typically the brightest followed by the apex and then the lateral wall. Infarcted myocardium will measure about 0–50 Hounsfield units. When measuring the Hounsfield unit level of the myocardium, use normal myocardium as an internal control within the same slice. Color mapping will likely be developed.

Hypoenhancement by CTA represents microvascular obstruction of blood flow. CTA, thus, looks at the interstitium of the myocardium. If a coronary stenosis is diagnosed, be sure to look at perfusion in the same territory to rule out infarction. The infarct area (region of hypoperfusion) will appear smaller than the delayed hyperenhancement region on MRI because in MRI the gadolinium is drawn into the interstitium of the myocardium and cannot escape, creating the appearance of a larger infarct area. CTA will underestimate the area of infarction by a factor of 10. An advantage of CTA, however, is that calcium in the myocardium can be seen whereas calcium is invisible on MRI.

Delayed hyperenhancement by CTA identifies infarcted territory with similar accuracy to MRI if the CT scan is repeated 15–20 minutes after the initial injection of contrast. The repeat scan may be performed at a lower energy level.

Future applications may include using cardiac CTA with adenosine stress to detect ischemia. Proof of concept has been published.[26]

Cardiac Function

Left ventricular function assessment permits the determination of left ventricular ejection fraction and also allows assessment of regional wall motion. Dual injection of contrast produces adequate right ventricular contrast enhancement to allow border detection of the right ventricular endocardium, thus permitting automated functional analysis of the right ventricle as well. Unlike echocardiography, for which multiple assumptions are necessary to accurately determine the ejection fraction (Simpson's rule), in CTA there are no geometric assumptions needed. Like echocardiography, wall thickening and not simply translational wall movement is used to assess function. Although functional analysis by CT has not been completely validated, it seems to be quite accurate. Using the dose modulation function does not preclude adequate functional analysis because the systolic radiation dose is high enough to allow accurate assessment of wall motion.

Many cardiac phases are required to evaluate ventricular function because capture of both end-systole and end-diastole is necessary. Generally, 10 to 20 phases are used for cardiac CTA whereas nuclear imaging uses eight phases and MRI uses 14–20 phases. A few simple steps (vender specific) by the technician are required to perform a functional analysis and the remainder is automated. Misregistration artifacts may produce artificial wall motion abnormalities. Increasing the slice thickness to around 5 mm will deemphasize these problems. However, by increasing the slice thickness, the image is blurred in the z-axis. Therefore, as mentioned previously, this approach is not sufficient for coronary analysis. Therefore, at least two datasets are generally reconstructed during the processing of a cardiac CTA. The first set (thin slices) is used to evaluate the coronary arteries and the second set (thick slices) is used for the functional analysis.

Using cardiac CTA for the assessment of ventricular function is a reasonable option for obese patients with poor echocardiographic windows. When doing this for the obese patient, use thick slices. Perform the noncontrasted CaSc first. If the CaSc is 0, then feel more comfortable that coronary lesions are not being overlooked (remember, the thicker the slice, the less detail one will see in the coronaries and thus lesions may be missed). Thicker slices create a larger voxel size and therefore less signal-to-noise ratio.

Assessing Calcium

A hypothesis yet to be proven is that calcium represents a healed atherosclerotic lesion. The critical coronary artery findings will often be in regions with soft plaque, often separate from the calcified areas. Do not be mesmerized

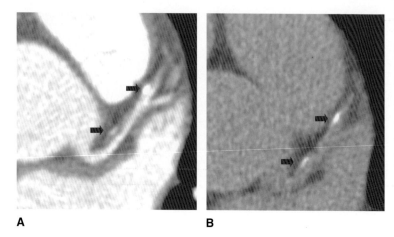

A   **B**

Figure 7.4. Calcium or plaque rupture. The potential importance of comparing the contrasted scan **(A)** with the noncontrasted scan **(B)**. Two bright densities are depicted by the black arrows on the contrast image in B. It is unclear whether these densities represent contrast in the arterial wall (plaque rupture) or calcium. By comparing with the noncontrasted scan in B, calcium is clearly seen in the identical regions, indicating that the findings on the contrasted scan represent calcium and not plaque rupture.

by the calcium. The true calcium area is always smaller (by a factor of 5 to 8) than what is seen because of volume rendering issues (sharing information from neighboring voxels) and partial volume effects. In essence, this occurs because of the limited spatial resolution of cardiac CTA. The calcium "bleeds" into the voxels to each side and above and below the center voxel. At the present time, the edge of the calcium is too small to be completely resolved. Therefore, calcium in one voxel will appear as though it occupies 5–8 voxels. The eye must be trained to accommodate this limitation.

Other clues may help assess the extent of the calcium. For example, the acoustic shadowing from the calcium should be no larger than the calcium itself. Dark areas larger than the area of the nearby calcium are more likely areas of soft plaque. Furthermore, density measurements may also serve as a guide (Hounsfield unit measurements). Beam hardening artifact will be negative numbers and soft plaque will be near +70). Finally, comparison with the noncontrasted scan will help assess if a bright area in the arterial wall is contrast (ulcerated lesion) or calcium (Figure 7.4). Calcium in the region of interest will be present on the noncontrasted scan.

Of clinical interest is that if the artery is rotated 360 degrees and lumen (dye) can be seen around or through the calcium, there is only a 2% chance of a hemodynamically significant lesion. If dye is not seen passing through the calcium, there is a 48% chance of a tight lesion (a flip of the coin) (Callister, The Tennessee Heart and Vascular Institute, unpublished oral communication, November 4, 2005). Some experts tend to label calcified lesions with visible lumen (no matter how small) as not flow limiting (Callister, The Tennessee Heart and Vascular Institute, unpublished oral communication, November 4, 2005). This approach will lead to high specificity. Others will grade the calcified lesion as potentially significant if the calcium covers >50% of the lumen (this approach will be very sensitive) (M. Poon, Cabrini Medical Center, New York, NY, unpublished oral communication, February 6, 2006). There is no absolutely correct approach and the individual reader must decide on his or her receiver operating curve (high specificity at the expense of sensitivity or vice versa).

Recognition of Artifacts

Because cardiac CTA involves imaging a moving structure and significant data reconstruction is required to form an image, many artifacts may be introduced into the final picture. It is imperative that these artifacts be recognized to avoid erroneous reads. In fact, abnormal findings should be considered artifact until proven otherwise. The following is a discussion of many common CTA artifacts.

Attenuation artifact (Figure 7.5) occurs because of a decreased signal-to-noise ratio and is often seen when imaging obese patients in whom the

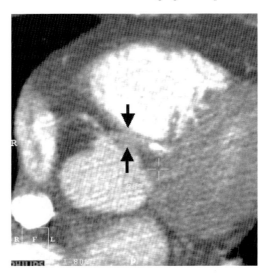

Figure 7.5. A good example of attenuation artifact. Note the grainy nature of the image caused by increased noise and decreased signal. Also note the anomalous left main coronary artery arising from the right coronary cusp and coursing between the aorta and the pulmonary artery (between the black arrows).

X-rays have difficulty penetrating. The image will appear grainy and may limit the ability to accurately diagnose coronary artery lesions.

Misregistration artifacts occur because of problems with collimation and image slab reconstruction in which the various slabs of data from different heartbeats are put together to recreate the entire image of the heart. Misregistration can occur from heart rate variability, patient movement, or breathing motion. Horizontal lines or seams in the image will be apparent where two image slabs do not match (Figure 7.6). Either the two image slabs are taken from different points in the cardiac cycle or the heart is physically in a different place when each of the two slabs is imaged. Recognizing the location of these pitfalls helps the reader to avoid attributing these problem areas to real lesions.

Misregistration from heart rate variability will be apparent on the image of the heart itself as steps throughout the entire length of the heart (Figure 7.7), whereas motion caused by breathing artifact will be noticeable as misregistration or misalignment from one slab to another best seen in the chest wall (Figure 7.8). Misregistration is more likely to be mistaken for a pseudo-lesion in thick MIP or VRT. Using thin MIP or MPR will help clarify the issue. Sometimes, despite great effort, it is impossible to figure out why an artifact is present. If so, try different reconstruction phases and see if it helps. If a certain slab of data is unreadable due to artifact, reconstruct it at 2% interval differences in either direction to see if that particular slab may be more optimally visualized. Furthermore, the slab may also be reconstructed using different reconstruction techniques and filters to optimize the image. With experience, artifacts will become easier to recognize even if the cause of the artifact is not clear.

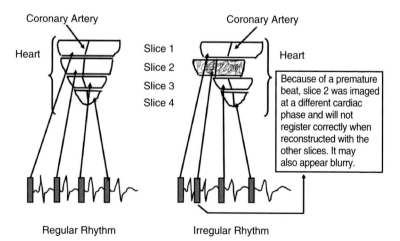

Figure 7.6. Cartoon depiction of a misregistration artifact in which slice 2 does not line up correctly with slices 1, 3, and 4 because it was imaged at a different cardiac phase from the remainder of the slices because of the irregular beat.

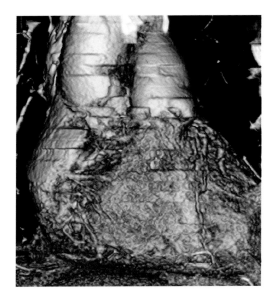

Figure 7.7. The typical step artifacts through the entire length of the heart typical for intrinsic cardiac motion. Notice that the step artifacts are seen generally throughout the whole heart and are not limited to one specific location.

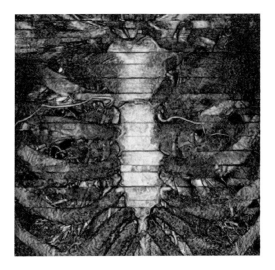

Figure 7.8. Misregistration along the length of the chest wall caused by breathing artifact.

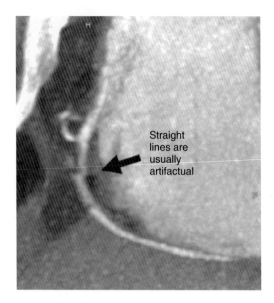

Straight
lines are
usually
artifactual

Figure 7.9. A straight-line misregistration artifact (black arrow) through the mid right coronary artery. Be wary of straight lines across the image because they are usually artifactual.

Always look at the axial MPR dataset because the axial MPR data are the true data and do not rely on registration of slices. Always scroll through the axial dataset to look for subtle jumps in the image while scrolling downward to assess for data loss or to confirm the validity of the dataset. Misregistration is minimized in the axial dataset. The coronal cuts and the sagittal cuts are the reconstruction datasets and are most susceptible to misregistration. With experience, readers can read around these artifacts and make diagnoses. If misregistration artifacts are seen in the sagittal or coronal planes, reading around them in the axial plane may be possible by taking advantage of the fact that no registration is needed in the axial plane.

When evaluating a problem area, clue in to the presence or absence of soft plaque. Atheroma must be present in some form or another for a lesion to be diagnosed. Be wary of straight lines on a cardiac CTA because they are likely artifacts (coronary dissections are very difficult to see because of the limits of spatial resolution) (Figure 7.9). In addition, rotating the vessel into the short axis will often help to differentiate a lesion from artifact.

Artifact caused by arrhythmia such as frequent premature contractions or other frequent ectopic beats will show up as a transverse artifact across the entire scan volume indicating a loss of data (Figure 7.10). Artifacts caused by cardiac motion itself will appear as step artifacts through the entire length of the heart and are not focal artifacts. It is possible to go back to the telemetry recordings at the scanner itself to analyze the heart rhythm for ectopic beats.

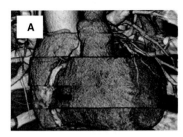
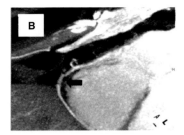

Figure 7.10. A. A typical rhythm artifact in which straight lines are seen through the heart but do not extend outside the heart itself into the surrounding tissue. The black arrows indicate the potential effect on coronary artery analysis. In the VRT image on the right (A), multiple misregistration artifacts are noted as the lines move through the artery. The black arrow demonstrates a blurred segment of the right coronary artery where this particular slab was imaged while the right coronary artery was rapidly moving. **B.** A displaced segment of the coronary artery (black arrow) resulting from the cardiac motion. Notice that the step artifact in this case is focal and limited to one location (black arrow).

In some systems, ectopy can sometimes be corrected by editing the electro-cardiographic tracing. Either a beat may be eliminated or the trigger may be moved to a different point in the cardiac cycle within a particular problematic R-R interval. Editing out too many beats, however, will produce too much data loss and exaggerate the line through the dataset. These are called banding artifacts (Figure 7.11) and appear as a thin, tubular line across the dataset and can be mistaken for a lesion if not recognized.

Intrinsic coronary artery motion will cause distinct artifacts as well. Blurriness will be introduced into the image. Motion can also cause distortion of the image often depicted as "twinning" (same structure is viewed twice in the

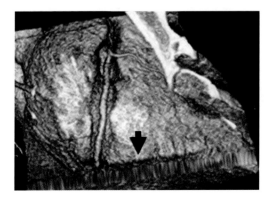

Figure 7.11. A typical banding artifact (black arrow) from data loss.

same image) or as a star or a set of wings (or some variant thereof) emanating from the artery (Figure 7.12). Blurring from motion can be seen in all planes (even axial) because it is a temporal resolution issue. If blurring is seen in the axial plane it must be the result of motion or ectopy but not misregistration. Knowing in advance the levels at which these blurring artifacts are seen will allow determination of whether a suspected lesion is actually artifact or real.

Beam hardening is another artifact that must be recognized and not mistaken for atheroma (Figure 7.13). This artifact occurs from attenuation of the X-ray beam by extremely dense structures such as metal (stents, pacemaker or defibrillator wires, sternal wires, vascular clips, Harrington rods, etc.) or calcium. Beam hardening artifact will demonstrate more negative Hounsfield units (< -50) whereas atheroma will be positive (around +70). Sharper kernels may help the reader interpret around dense objects. Use thin MIP or MPR and dial the window level down to see inside stents or around calcium or clips or metal artifacts.

Realize that lesions are overestimated in bends or tortuous regions. A stenosis at a bend is probably not significant. Significant stenoses rarely occur in these locations but rather occur more frequently at branch points. It is far more likely that an apparent abnormality at a bend is attributable to streaming of dye and not to a true stenosis.

Branch points can also create the appearance of a pseudo-lesion. It is very important to rotate a vessel around in 360 degrees to visualize a problem area in two orthogonal planes before making a diagnosis. In most cases, this will lay out the branch vessel eliminating the appearance of a pseudo-lesion.

The "windmill" artifact is frequently seen when the ECG lead is misplaced over the heart during the scan. This artifact is easily recognizable.

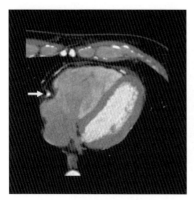 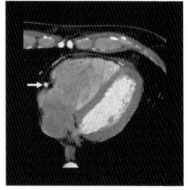

A   **B**

Figure 7.12. The typical "wings" that emanate from a coronary artery (in this case the right coronary artery, white arrow on **A**) when intrinsic coronary motion is seen. **B.** This image shows the right coronary artery, in the same location, as a uniform circle (short axis, white arrow) and demonstrates no motion artifact. **B** was taken from a more optimal phase.

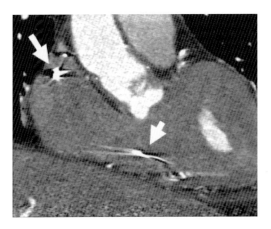

Figure 7.13. Typical beam hardening artifacts (white arrows) caused by pacing wires in the right atrium and right ventricle.

Assessment for Ancillary Radiologic Findings

Figures 7.14–7.18 depict the normal noncardiac axial plane anatomy. Whereas most cardiologists will have a radiologist over-read their studies for ancillary findings, others do not (see discussion below). Having some knowl-

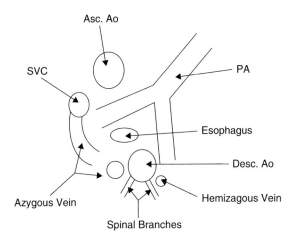

Figure 7.14. Typical axial plane anatomy at the level of the pulmonary artery (PA) bifurcation. Asc. Ao, ascending aorta; SVC, superior vena cava; Desc. Ao, descending aorta.

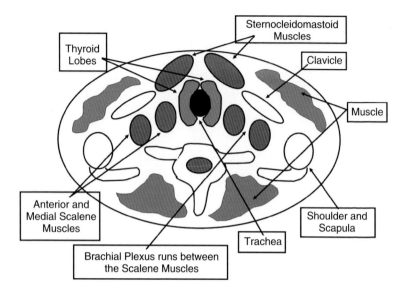

Figure 7.15. Normal axial plane anatomy at the level of the thyroid gland. Notice the area between the scalene muscles where the brachial plexus resides.

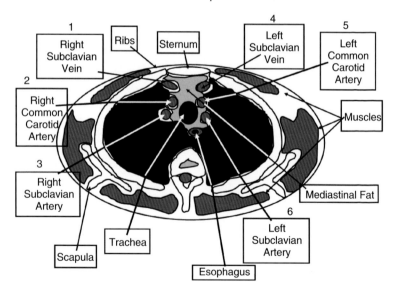

Figure 7.16. Normal axial anatomy just above the aortic arch. Note the six arterial outlines (numbered 1–6). Lymph nodes and masses may be found here. If more than the six arterial outlines are seen, pathology exists.

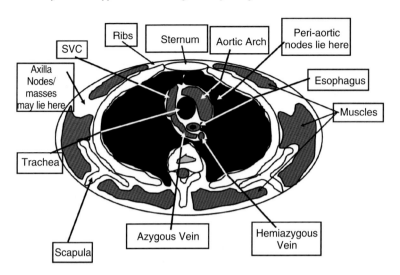

Figure 7.17. Normal axial anatomy at the level of the aortic arch. Give particular attention to the periaortic region where lymph nodes may reside. In addition, examine the axilla. Lymph nodes and masses may be present in these areas. SVC, superior vena cava.

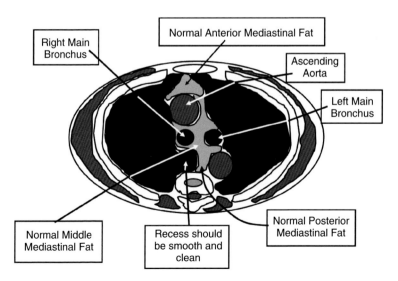

Figure 7.18. Normal axial anatomy at the level of the aorta before the arch. Note the subtracheal recess (white asterisk). This space should be smooth. If blunted, pathology is present.

edge in this area is critical. With some experience, the cardiologist may easily diagnose basic ancillary findings.

Be sure to systematically evaluate the mediastinal windows, giving particular attention to the soft tissue. The centerline for the mediastinal window is +40. At the level of the thyroid (Figure 7.15), give attention to the size of the thyroid gland and to possible mediastinal masses. In addition, note that the brachial plexus runs between the scalene muscles. Just above the aortic arch (Figure 7.16) reside the six circular outlines of the aortic arch branch vessels and veins. These vessels are the left subclavian artery, left subclavian vein, left common carotid artery, right subclavian artery, right subclavian vein, and right common carotid artery. Densities other than the six structures mentioned above represent lymph nodes or masses. In general, lymph nodes are pathologic if they are not calcified and >1.5 cm in size.

At the level of the aortic arch (Figure 7.17), look in the axillary regions for lymph nodes and masses. Give attention to the breast tissue to exclude breast masses. In addition, evaluate the mediastinum for anterior (in front of the heart), middle (even with the heart), and posterior (behind the heart) mediastinal masses. Anterior mediastinal masses are thymomas, thyroid tumors, teratomas, or lymphomas. There should be no pathologic lymph nodes in the mediastinum or in the periaortic area.

Assess the inferior vena cava, superior vena cava, and azygous vein (Figure 7.17) and understand the pertinent anatomy. The inferior and superior mesenteric veins along with the splenic vein drain into the portal vein. The portal vein routes blood from the capillary beds of the intestines to the capillary beds of the liver. The renal veins empty into the inferior vena cava. The azygous vein receives blood from the veins from parts of the chest wall, esophagus and right lung and mediastinum. The azygous vein is also the collateral route to the inferior vena cava from the superior vena cava. Note the extent of the fat around the superior vena cava. Too much adipose tissue in this area may constrict the superior vena cava. This phenomenon is also associated with atrial septal fat and dysrhythmias. Assess the size of the superior vena cava and inferior vena cava. Furthermore, increased contrast inside a large inferior vena cava probably represents significant tricuspid regurgitation and increased right-sided pressures.

Evaluate the esophagus, which lies behind the trachea (Figures 7.16 and 7.17). Hiatal hernias are easily seen and appear as a region with multiple black spots just above the diaphragm in the location of the esophagus. The esophagus should appear as a small single black circle. In addition, assess the liver, the kidneys, and the adrenal glands.

Give particular attention to the lungs using the lung window. The center of the lung window is −500 Hounsfield units. Failure to carefully evaluate the lungs will cause the reader to overlook possible significant lung pathology such as nodules, masses, infiltrates, adenopathy, and scarring. Pathologic nodules should not be missed. Calcified nodules are benign and likely represent old granulomatous disease whereas noncalcified nodules are more concerning. By returning to the mediastinal window, calcified lesions may be distinguished from noncalcified abnormalities.

Note that in many CTA scans, lung nodules will be identified. Usually slow-growing, less aggressive neoplasms are picked up in the early stages. In addition, less than 1% of all nodules are cancerous and wedge resection carries a 3% mortality rate and is accompanied by significant pain and morbidity.[27] There is a 99% false-positive rate on these nodules and only 1%–2% are neoplastic.[27] Performing radiologic follow-up on these small nodules increases healthcare cost, radiation exposure, and patient and doctor anxiety for no apparent patient benefit. Patients who are appropriately screened for lung cancer are generally patients who are older and at higher risk. Scans for lung cancer screening utilize a larger sFOV. In addition, thicker slices are used.

There is debate on whether radiologists should generally over-read cardiac CTA studies. Local standard of care principles may serve as a guide in this area. These authors believe that radiologists and cardiologists must collaborate to create a successful cardiac CTA program.

The Fleischner Society[27] reports that nodules ≤4 mm are low risk and require no follow-up. The Fleischner Society also recommends that nodules >4–6 mm in patients at high risk should be followed up with a repeat CT scan in 6 months and if no change, another scan should be obtained 18–24 months later, and if no change, no follow-up is necessary thereafter.[27] In low-risk patients with nodules of >4–6 mm, a 12-month repeat scan is indicated.[27] If no change, no further scanning is necessary.[27] If a nodule is spiculated with irregular borders, it must be pursued promptly.

When examining the lungs, do not overlook the pleura and be sure to rule out pleural effusions. Also, be aware of the typical ground-glass appearance. This represents early air space disease (adult respiratory distress syndrome, hypersensitivity pneumonitis, or drug toxicity).

Be cognizant of the hypogenetic lung syndrome (scimitar syndrome). This is a congenital anomaly consisting of hypoplasia of the right lung and of the right pulmonary artery as well. There is also partial or total anomalous venous return from the right lung into the systemic veins (usually the inferior vena cava). If severe, the pulmonary artery can arise from the aorta. The radiologic findings are a small hemithorax, a mediastinal shift to the right side, a small right hilum, and anomalous venous return.

Examine the trachea for lesions such as polyps, mucous plugs, or tumors and understand the anatomy of the bronchi noting any bronchial and peribronchial lesions as well as possible external bronchial compression. The anatomy of the bronchi is as follows (Figure 7.19). The left main stem bronchus gives rise to the left upper lobe bronchus and the left lower lobe bronchus. The left upper lobe bronchus branches into the apical posterior segment, the anterior segment, and the lingular segment. The left lower lobe bronchus gives rise to the superior and basal segments. The right main stem bronchus branches into the right upper lobe bronchus, the right middle lobe bronchus, and the right lower lobe bronchus. The right upper lobe bronchus gives rise to the superior, anterior, and posterior segments. The right middle lobe bronchus gives rise to medial and lateral segments. From the right lower lobe bronchus emanates the superior segment and the anterior, medial, lateral, and posterior segments. Lesions in the lungs are located based on the bronchial anatomy. At

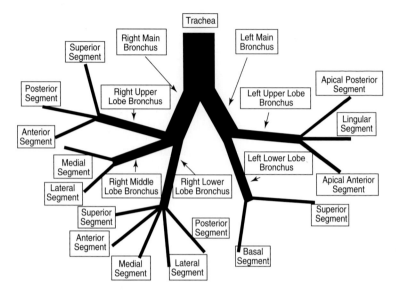

Figure 7.19.   Illustration of the normal bronchial tree anatomy, which helps to localize lesions found in the lungs.

the level of the right and left main bronchi is a smooth recess (Figure 7.18). Abnormal tissue (infiltrate, lymph node, or a mass) will blunt this area. Pathology in this region should not be overlooked. In addition, do not overlook subcarinal masses.

Be aware of other congenital anomalies such as mediastinal cysts. Multiple types of mediastinal cysts exist. Bronchogenic cysts arise from primitive bronchi. They contain fluid of variable viscosity, which can be dense (from water density to denser than muscle). Most are located along the right paratracheal wall or near the carina in the middle or posterior mediastinum. They are usually in contact with the carina and may slightly deform the carina. Duplication cysts arise from the primitive foregut. They are usually in the posterior mediastinum in a paraspinal location. They are most often connected to the esophagus. Other than location, their appearance is indistinguishable from bronchogenic cysts. Neurenteric cysts are connected to the meninges through a defect in one or more vertebral bodies. They are rarely connected to the esophagus. Pleuropericardial cysts are most often in the cardiophrenic angles or lower aspect of the pericardium. The differential diagnosis of a mediastinal cyst is an abscess (abscesses do not calcify), old hematomas (may calcify), cystic tumors, and congenital lesions such as cystic lymphangiomas. Pericardial cysts may also be seen and are usually right sided.

Finally, the bones should be viewed in the bone window. Degenerative joint disease may be seen. In severe cases, there may be air inside the bone known as the vacuum phenomenon. Neural tumors may also be seen. Harrington rods may be identified. Spinal stimulator catheters can be visualized as well.

Reporting

In general, the CTA report should prove useful to the referring physician. It should include patient identification data, a brief clinical history, and the test indication. The specific question asked should be documented. A brief description of the procedural technique should be included. This section should comment on the type of scanner, the collimation and resolution data, the scan field, the contrast amount and type, the contrast injection location and protocol, the premedication used, the radiation dose and scan protocol (dose modulation, etc.), and the power of the scan in mAs. This information will help with reimbursement and with documentation of patient data and radiation. Also include information about the reconstruction and analysis techniques, such as phases, filters used, and whether or not functional analysis was performed (currently and add on code).

The section on findings should include a comment on scan quality. Note artifacts and make disclaimers about the usefulness of the scan information based on the quality so that the referring physician will have an idea of the reliability of the test. Note that 6%–20% of scans are unreadable (Callister, The Tennessee Heart and Vascular Institute, unpublished oral communication, November 4, 2005). Describe specific arterial segments that cannot be evaluated and report the reason. Comment on motion, arrhythmias, contrast quality, and scan timing. Report the CaSc and clinical significance. Report the coronary artery findings and graft findings if applicable. Always comment on perfusion. In addition, report on morphology including the mitral and aortic valve structure, the cardiac chamber sizes, the presence or absence of shunts, the left atrial appendage, and the great vessels and pulmonary arteries. If clinically pertinent, comment on the pulmonary and cardiac veins and the pericardium. Finally, include a section for the radiology ancillary findings.

When assessing for atherosclerosis, describe the extent (focal, diffuse, limited, etc.) and location of the plaque. Describe whether there is calcified plaque, mixed plaque, or soft plaque. When discussing the coronary and or graft findings, comment generally on the size of arteries and bypass grafts. Always make an effort to grade the stenoses in clinically relevant and useful terms. Grades such as mild, moderate, and severe are not clinically useful because these gradations do not help with the clinical decision of whether cardiac catheterization, stress testing, or medical therapy alone is indicated. However, grading a stenosis too specifically may be misleading, because the spatial resolution of coronary CTA is not good enough to exactly grade a lesion. A useful rule is to group lesion severities into general, clinically relevant categories such as mild, mild to moderate, moderate, moderate to severe, and severe. Alternatively, quartile gradations may be used such as 0%–25%, 25%–50%, 50%–75%, and 75%–90%. Always underestimate the severity of a calcified lesion unless no contrast is seen going through it. Remember that the calcium appears to be 5–8 times larger than its true area (blooming artifact).

Clarification terms such as "not flow limiting," "potentially flow limiting," or "probably flow limiting" may be useful. In addition, using a statement such as "cannot be excluded" is reasonable; for example, "a severe flow-limiting stenosis cannot be excluded." A word such as "patent" is often used to describe a stent or bypass graft if the region is open but in-stent restenosis or the graft anastomosis cannot be seen well. Remember, subtotal occlusions and complete occlusions with collateral filling of the distal vessel are indistinguishable since collateral vessels are most often not visualized by CTA.

Be honest about what cannot be assessed such as distal arteries, plaque inside smaller stents, and graft regions obscured by clips. Describe why the area could not be further characterized such as poor contrast or artifact. Terms such as "limited study" with descriptors may be useful. A statement such as "the artery is probably free of significant stenoses but motion artifact limits analysis" may be needed. The reader must be comfortable with approximations and with doing the best that can be done and with being honest about these limitations in the report. Remember that answering the question is the most important goal. Do not waste time or energy on minute details that are unimportant since collateral vessels.

The impression should be concise, specific, and to the point. Summarize the findings and answer the specific question asked. Comment on the reliability of the findings and the limitations of the findings based on scan quality. Provide a comment on the reasonable next steps (medical therapy for risk factor control, stress testing, catheterization, cardiology consultation, etc.). The report should be useful to the referring physician. Images of the important findings may be included in the final report, which serves to inform the ordering physician and to document the findings.

Using clinical decision theory (Table 7.1) as a guide to the potential next step is important. Indicating that a cardiac CTA is "high risk" is reasonable.

Table 7.1. A possible algorithm to guide clinical decision theory after a cardiac CTA

	Normal CTA	+CTA (low risk)	+CTA (high risk)
Anginal pain	Nuclear scan (often will be normal) for reassurance	Nuclear scan and medications	Cardiac catheterization
Nonanginal pain	Reassurance	Medical treatment	Cardiac catheterization (because almost always a tight lesion). Nuclear scan is also acceptable.

High-risk findings include left ventricular dysfunction, moderate or extensive mixed lesions (calcified and soft plaque), large or totally circumferential calcified lesions in which no contrast gets through, and visibly tight soft plaque lesions. Remember that lesions at cardiac catheterization more closely mimic the soft plaque CTA lesion and not the calcified one.

8. Specific Applications and Useful Clinical Pearls

Atypical Chest Pain in the Emergency Room

More than 6 million patients in the United States present to the emergency room (ER) per year with chest pain.[28] A significant amount of money is wasted on inappropriate chest pain evaluations and admissions. Many patients are mistakenly sent home with acute coronary syndromes and still others are unnecessarily admitted to the hospital for noncardiac, minor chest pain. The key point is that the clinical presentation is not perfect in triaging the patients with chest pain in the ER. The evaluation of chest pain in the ER needs to improve.

With 16-slice computed tomographic angiography (CTA), the negative predictive value for the diagnosis of significant coronary artery disease is approximately 93%–100%. This test would most benefit the intermediate-probability patients in the ER. These patients would include those with a clinically reasonable presentation, and a normal or equivocal electrocardiogram (ECG) with negative cardiac markers and two or more cardiovascular risk factors. Gaspar et al.[20] illustrated that by using cardiac CTA, hospitalization could be aborted in 33% of the patients presenting to the ER with chest pain.

By the same token, there are logistical concerns with this approach. Twenty-four hour coverage would be necessary to provide urgent expert readings. In addition, patient preparation is cumbersome and requires significant expertise that may be difficult to obtain during evening hours. Furthermore, at the present time, 4%–15% of coronary segments are unable to be visualized in the elective patient undergoing CTA and the number of segments that cannot be visualized would be expected to increase in the emergency setting. All segments must be visualized to comfortably clear an ER patient for discharge in the setting of a suspected acute coronary syndrome.

Scanner availability may also be an issue if the scanner is occupied with other ER patients. In addition, there are still few data supporting the use of cardiac CTA for the "triple rule out" and for suspected acute coronary syndromes in the ER. It is also certain that calcium scoring is inappropriate in the symptomatic patient.

One must keep in mind that physiology is not always connected to anatomy and that coronary physiology and not coronary anatomy is the best determinant of outcome and prognosis. As such, a potentially non–flow-limiting lesion may still be an unstable lesion. There is far more literature to support the use of nuclear stress testing in the ER setting and, therefore, the routine use of cardiac CTA in the ER setting may be premature.

Bypass Graft Analysis

Cardiac CTA may be used to assess bypass graft patency as well as to evaluate the patient undergoing repeat bypass surgery. In the latter case, the CTA examination is used to identify the location of a previously utilized left or right internal mammary artery (LIMA or RIMA, respectively). For example, if the LIMA is adhered to the chest wall, repeat bypass surgery may be more difficult and require additional planning. Knowledge of this anatomy before surgery may be helpful.

It is particularly important to use the right antecubital vein for contrast injection in bypass patients because injection of the left antecubital vein will necessitate that contrast cross over the chest on its way to the heart, potentially obstructing visualization of sections of the bypass graft anatomy. In addition, in bypass patients, the contrast volume must be increased to assure adequate contrast throughout the scan.

As a general overview, begin by viewing the chest wall. In addition to observing for breathing artifacts as discussed previously, examining the chest wall in the coronal or even the axial planes will permit the reader to determine if the left internal mammary (LIMA) and or right internal mammary artery (RIMA) were used for bypass (Figure 8.1). If these arteries remain in their normal anatomic positions, one need not search for them as bypass grafts. In addition, examining the chest wall will exclude sternal malunion and sternal wire fractures. Furthermore, in the axial short axis view at the level of the pulmonary artery bifurcation, the number of grafts can be counted because they are usually seen in this region in short axis. In the axial plane, the right coronary artery (RCA) graft arises from the aorta at the 11 o'clock position. The left anterior descending (LAD) artery graft is most often seen in short axis at 2 o'clock whereas the circumflex and obtuse marginal grafts are located in short axis at 4 o'clock.

The graft closest to the aortic valve is usually the saphenous vein graft (SVG) to the RCA system. Moving superiorly, the next graft will be the SVG to the obtuse marginal branches or to the circumflex artery. The most superior graft is generally to the LAD or diagonal system.

Image reconstruction protocols for bypass surgery patients may be somewhat different than those used for the assessment of the coronary arteries alone. Cases encompassing bypass grafts are often reconstructed in two sections. Section one includes a selected field of view (sFOV) to encompass the proximal anastemosis and body of the grafts. This would cover the lung apices to the proximal ascending aorta for an LIMA and would include the mid-ascending aorta to the proximal ascending aorta for vein grafts. Since this region of the bypass grafts exhibit little intrinsic motion, this section need only be reconstructed in one optimal phase to save computer storage space and time. Multiphasic analysis is then performed (limited sFOV) from the mid-aorta to the diaphragm to allow better assessment of the native coronaries, of the distal bypass grafts, and of the anastomotic sites.

In patients with LIMA conduits, some suggest reducing the sFOV so as not to include the apex of the lung where the ostium of the LIMA is located.

The advantages to this approach are that less radiation is used (for each 1 cm of scan field there is an associated 1 mSv of radiation) and there is less required breath hold thus increasing the likelihood for diagnostic quality images at the distal anastomotic sites. This approach is controversial because, although rare, problems can be seen at the LIMA ostium. Furthermore, sub-clavian stenoses that may compromise blood flow to the LIMA should be excluded.

If the LIMA is not visualized at all and a patent native vessel is seen, note only that the LIMA may be atretic. Do not report the LIMA to be occluded in this case because competitive flow from the native vessel as the cause for the lack of visualization of the LIMA cannot be excluded. To visualize the entire LIMA, use a higher contrast volume (up to 120 cc).

To read a bypass study, start from the volume rendering technique (VRT) images to get a general overview. The cut plane function may be quite useful (vender specific). With this technique, the VRT image may be cut away in layers using the mouse to remove overlapping structures. This technique may aid with orientation in complicated bypass graft cases. Look at the chest wall for abnormalities and to identify whether the LIMA and or RIMA are used as conduits. In addition, a general orientation of graft number, location, and patency may be obtained. Bypass graft stumps may be identified, which represent occluded grafts. Stumps should not be confused with pledgets. Pledgets have a typical wrinkled appearance whereas stumps are smooth (Figure 8.2). In addition, because pledgets are placed in the region of the aortic vent, they are generally located high on the ascending aorta near the aortic arch. Bypass grafts are not usually seen in this location.

The coronal plane is excellent for evaluating bypass grafts. Start by coming anteriorly to the sternum. Widen the maximal intensity projection (MIP) to >5 mm and open up the window width to increase the number of shades of gray. The LIMA and RIMA will then be seen in their normal anatomic positions and if one or the other or both are absent, it was used for grafting (Figure 8.1). If the LIMA and RIMA are not used, look at the diameter of each and they should be equal. Follow this with an assessment of the sternum (sternal malunion or sternal wire fracture). Progress posteriorly through the imaging planes until the heart is seen. In the coronal view as the planes move posteriorly, the RCA graft is first seen, followed by the LIMA. The body of the LIMA is best seen in the coronal view but the distal anastomosis is best seen in the sagittal view. Moving further posteriorly, the grafts to the left circulation will then be visualized.

Often, an arterial free graft such as a free RIMA graft or a free radial graft may be distinguished from an SVG by the absence of clips. In addition, the diameter of these free arterial grafts is similar to a LIMA whereas vein grafts are larger in diameter.

Be sure to adequately evaluate the native coronary arteries distal to the bypass graft anastomoses to exclude lesions beyond the anastomotic points and to identify unprotected native branch vessels. If an artery beyond the distal anastomosis has more contrast than proximal to the anastomosis, the graft is probably patent.

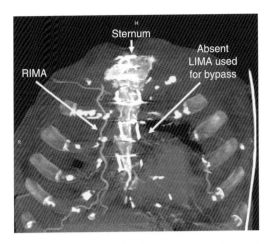

Figure 8.1. The chest wall in MIP where the RIMA is visualized and the LIMA is absent indicating that the LIMA was used for bypass grafting.

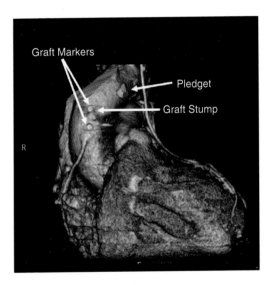

Figure 8.2. The typical appearance of an occluded bypass graft stump versus a pledget. The pledget is higher on the aorta and wrinkled whereas the stump is smooth and resides in a typical location for a bypass graft (in this case between two graft markers). Note the patent RCA graft and the patent LIMA. This one VRT image provides an excellent, rapid overview of the bypass graft anatomy.

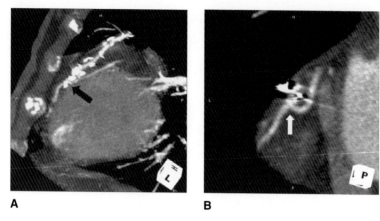

A   **B**

Figure 8.3. Examples of two separate bypass graft anastomoses. The anastomosis in **(A)** (black arrow) is an example of an LIMA grafted to the LAD artery. Here, the anastomosis is not well seen because of the presence of multiple vascular clips. The image in **(B)** depicts an SVG to the obtuse marginal (OM) branch and here, the anastomosis (white arrow) is fortuitously seen because the vascular clips were placed above the anastomotic site.

Clips may often create challenges in assessing bypass grafts because of beam-hardening artifact and their potential to obscure the graft lumen or anastomosis point. Very thin MIP, oblique multiplanar reformatting (MPR), and curved MPR are the best options to read around vascular clips. Sharp filters may also help. Finally, rotating 360 degrees around the artery may help in finding an angle to adequately assess the lumen. Sometimes, however, bypass clips preclude assessment of the lumen and this must be reported as a limitation of the study.

Figure 8.3 depicts an anastomosis obscured by a large number of vascular clips and another anastomosis that is well visualized. One cannot predict which of the previous examples will be present in a specific patient.

Evaluation of Coronary Stents

Cardiac CTA is not optimal for the general evaluation of coronary stents because the spatial resolution is not quite good enough to reliably visualize the intrastent lumen. Thus, CTA should not be routinely used for the evaluation of coronary stents if the stent is the primary clinical question. Having said this, there are instances in which stents may be assessable. Stents >3.5–4.0 mm may be adequately assessed. In addition, Velocity and NIR stents are almost invisible by CTA and are thus easily assessed. Cypher stents are more difficult to evaluate by CTA and Taxus stents are the worst.

To adequately visualize a stent lumen, use adequate power (mAs) to minimize noise. Limiting patient motion and breathing is crucial and it is particularly important that the heart rhythm be steady and slow with little variability. Sharp reconstruction filters are best to see within the stent (Figure 8.4). These filters will minimize the blooming artifact from the stent metal, which limits the ability to see inside the stent. Also, emphasize stent struts by widening the window width to bring down the background brightness. In addition, thin MIP and MPR are best for stent analysis (similar to vascular clips and other forms of metal). VRT is inappropriate for the stent evaluation.

A focal dark area within a stent is usually a real in-stent lesion whereas uniform midlevel gray inside the stent usually represents a patent stent without significant in-stent stenoses. A focal dark region in a stent should not be attributed to beam-hardening artifact because beam hardening would not be caused by just a region of struts but rather would be seen resulting from all struts (diffuse blackness within the stent). Rotating around the stent may help in analyzing within the stent and this may be performed manually or by using curved MPR. Note that plaque in regions just before and just after a stent (stent borders) is often overemphasized and lesions appear tighter than they really are. If no contrast is seen within the stent but the artery is visualized distally, one cannot distinguish between a subtotal occlusion of the stent with a trickling of dye going through the stent versus a complete occlusion and distal filling via collaterals.

Sometimes it is difficult to differentiate a stent from calcium especially when the typical strut appearance is not evident. In these instances, measure the Hounsfield units of the region of interest. A stent will have units typical for metal (>1000). The density of calcium is much lower.

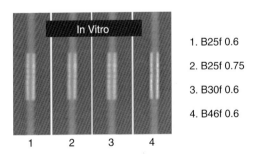

1. B25f 0.6

2. B25f 0.75

3. B30f 0.6

4. B46f 0.6

Figure 8.4. A CT image of an in vitro stent using progressively sharper convolution filters (1–4). Note that the clarity of the image inside the stent improves markedly as sharper filters are used. The sharpest filter (B46f 0.6) provides the most clarity inside the stent.

Assessment of Heart Valves

To evaluate the heart valves, the slice thickness needs to be as thin as possible to optimize visualization of fine structures. For the aortic valve, find the end systolic reconstruction where the valve is maximally opened. Then create a short axis of the valve with the maximum orifice size. The number of leaflets may be identified (tricuspid versus bicuspid). If a bicuspid valve is identified, be sure to rule out a concomitant aortic aneurysm and or a coarctation of the aorta. Aortic valve calcification is also easily seen and correlates with the degree of stenosis.[16] If the calcium score of the aortic valve is >400, an echocardiogram should be obtained to rule out significant aortic stenosis.[16] If indicated, planimetry is performed to evaluate valve area. Significant blurring from motion artifact may preclude accurate planimetry. Valvular masses, thrombi, and vegetations (Figure 8.5) may be visualized. The density of the object (Hounsfield units) can also be measured to help characterize the tissue or the mass, although differentiating the three from one another may be challenging. Ring abscesses may also be seen.

The mitral valve may also be analyzed in great detail. Mitral annular calcification and leaflet abnormalities may be seen. Masses, thrombi, vegetations (Figure 8.5), and abscesses may be visualized. Mitral valve prolapse and mitral

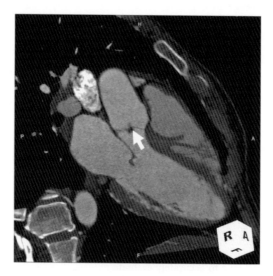

Figure 8.5. An aortic valve vegetation (white arrow). This would be difficult to pick up in the absence of contrast because the CT density of the vegetation is similar to normal tissue. The clinical picture would usually provide a clue.

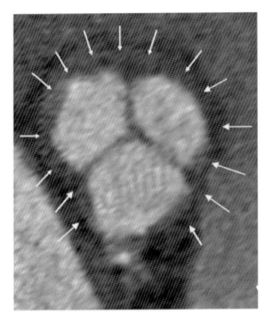

Figure 8.6. An aortic valve bioprosthesis. Note that the valve ring is well visualized (white arrows) and demonstrates the same CT density as the normal surrounding tissue.

stenosis may be identified. Systolic anterior motion of the mitral valve or of the chordae tendineae may also be seen. The valve should be assessed in short axis as well as in the two- and three-chamber views.

Although the tricuspid and pulmonary valves are not well visualized by cardiac CT, significant contrast in the inferior vena cava may imply significant tricuspid regurgitation.

Bioprosthetic valves may be well visualized. The valve ring has the same CT density as normal tissue (Figure 8.6). In addition, mechanical valves are also well visualized (Figure 8.7). Cinefluoroscopy is also an excellent technique to evaluate the function of prosthetic mechanical valves. Narrow the window down to permit more precise visualization of the valve and create the appropriate imaging plane to accurately evaluate motion. A real-time cine loop of multiple phases may be played to evaluate leaflet motion and to rule out clot and pannus. This technique may be more effective than fluoroscopy. Thicker MIP may be needed to better visualize mechanical valves.

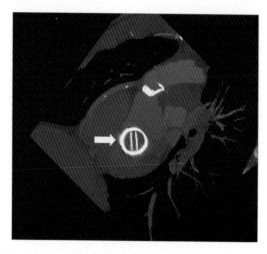

Figure 8.7. A St. Jude mechanical mitral valve during diastole (white arrow). The leaflets are open. Viewing this valve in cine mode (cinefluoroscopy) is an excellent method to assess mechanical prosthetic valve function.

Electrophysiology Applications

There are two main electrophysiology applications for cardiac CTA: The pre- and postassessment of atrial fibrillation ablation patients and evaluation of cardiac venous anatomy in the potential cardiac resynchronization therapy patient.

For the potential atrial fibrillation ablation patient, CTA is used to characterize the pulmonary veins (location, size, anomalies). The ostia of the pulmonary veins can be measured in orthogonal short-axis planes. Here the axial and coronal planes are used to create a short-axis view of each pulmonary vein in the sagittal section to measure the ostium of the pulmonary veins. This will also help size the lasso catheter, which is used for the ablation procedure. Anomalous pulmonary venous return must be excluded. Furthermore, CTA is used to size the left atrium, to exclude atrial thrombi (Figure 8.8), and to exclude atrial masses. In addition, the interatrial septum must be characterized (lipomatous hypertrophy) because a transseptal approach is necessary. Finally, the anatomic relationship of the esophagus to the pulmonary veins should be defined to help the electrophysiologist define the risk of a pulmonary vein to esophagus fistula formation as a result of the ablation procedure.

Pulmonary venous anatomy may be highly variable. The order of accuracy for assessing pulmonary venous anatomy is as follows: CTA > intracardiac echo > transesophageal echocardiography (TEE) > venography. CTA is the most sensitive because one can manipulate the image in all angles and planes.

In addition, intracardiac echo often underestimates the ostia of the pulmonary veins. Forty percent of patients have anatomic variations in their pulmonary venous anatomy and only 60% of people have only four pulmonary veins.[29] Accessory veins (present in up to 33% of patients) place one at higher risk for atrial fibrillation.[29] Accessory pulmonary veins are usually right sided.[29] Conjoined veins are less common (10%). These are usually left sided (88%).[29] Figure 8.9 illustrates common variations in pulmonary venous anatomy. The left superior pulmonary vein is the most common source for atrial fibrillation (40%–60%).[29]

The protocol used to evaluate the coronary arteries is also used to visualize the left atrium, left atrial appendage, and pulmonary veins. Reconstruction is performed in one phase (60%–70% will do). Practically any single phase will do because the atrium is no longer contracting when atrial fibrillation is present. No less than 100 cc of contrast is needed and the study need not be gated. The timing of the scan for pulmonary venous imaging is not critical. It may, however, be timed a bit earlier than that for coronary evaluation.

CTA may also be used in routine follow-up after atrial fibrillation ablation to screen for pulmonary vein stenosis and thrombosis, which is usually seen in the right inferior pulmonary vein and usually occurs in <6 months. Therefore, the first postablation CTA should be done at 6 months. Pulmonary vein stenosis may cause cough, hemoptysis, shortness of breath, and pulmonary infarction.

CTA may also be used to assess the cardiac venous anatomy in preparation for cardiac resynchronization therapy (biventricular pacing). The same technique used for visualizing the coronary arteries may be used to visualize the

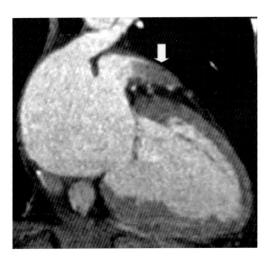

Figure 8.8. A good example of a left atrial appendage thrombus. The density of the thrombus would measure approximately +50 Hounsfield units.

cardiac veins. However, the timing of the scan is delayed to allow venous filling (trigger the scan 6 seconds after the peak of the contrast bolus). CTA overcomes the shortcomings of catheter coronary sinus venography. Cardiac CTA is rapid, safe, and reliable for this application. It will save fluoroscopy time and multiple contrast injections required for less-effective coronary sinus venography and it is noninvasive. In addition, unlike venography, CTA will display three-dimensional anatomy. However, CTA may be limited in sicker patients who are dyspneic with limited ability to β-block.

The cardiac venous anatomy may also be correlated with left ventricular scarring and regional wall thickening. This evaluation will permit prior assessment of whether a percutaneous left-sided lead will be effective. In addition, the probability of diaphragmatic stimulation with the left ventricular lead may be predicted. Finally, the thebesian valve may be visualized (coronary sinus valve remnant), which may prevent cannulation of the coronary sinus. If after a thorough evaluation of the cardiac venous anatomy, the electrophysiologist believes a percutaneous approach will be suboptimal, the surgeon can place a thoracoscopic left ventricular lead.

The coronary venous system (Figure 8.10) is more variable than the coronary arterial system. Typically, the veins are associated with the coronary arteries and are larger than the coronary arteries. The coronary sinus is a wide venous channel 9–10 mm in diameter. The coronary sinus starts at a confluence with the vein of Marshall, which drains the atrium and runs obliquely along the back of the left atrium. The coronary sinus drains into the right atrium through the thebesian valve at the right atrial junction. The great cardiac vein drains into the coronary sinus via the valve of Vieussens. The great cardiac vein runs with the circumflex and receives branches from the left

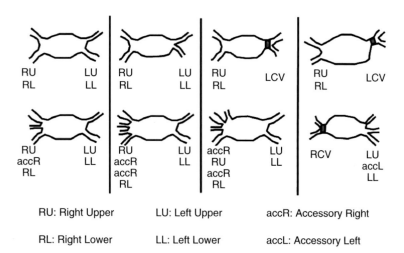

RU: Right Upper   LU: Left Upper   accR: Accessory Right

RL: Right Lower   LL: Left Lower   accL: Accessory Left

Figure 8.9. Cartoon drawing of the common variations in pulmonary venous anatomy.

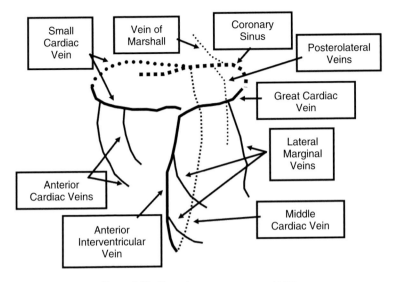

Figure 8.10. Normal coronary venous anatomy.

atrium, left ventricle, and right ventricle. There are also lateral marginal veins that empty into the great cardiac vein and drain the lateral left ventricular arteries. The lateral marginal veins are favorite targets for cardiac resynchronization therapy.

The anterior interventricular vein runs with the LAD artery and starts at the cardiac apex and also drains into the great cardiac vein. The middle cardiac vein runs posteriorly with the posterior descending artery and receives branches from the left and right ventricle. The middle cardiac vein is an occasional resynchronization target. The small cardiac vein travels with the RCA and drains the right ventricular arteries. The small cardiac vein empties into the coronary sinus. The posterior vein of the left ventricle travels with the distal circumflex along the diaphragmatic surface. It is an alternate target for cardiac resynchronization leads. The anterior cardiac veins drain the ventral right ventricle. Smallest coronary veins (veins of thebesius) are minute veins that start in the myocardium and empty into the atria and rarely into the ventricles.

Evaluation of the Aorta

The normal anatomy of the aorta is depicted in Figure 8.11. Common pathology of the aorta includes aneurysms, dissections, atherosclerosis, calcification (note that there is often a small amount of focal calcification at the

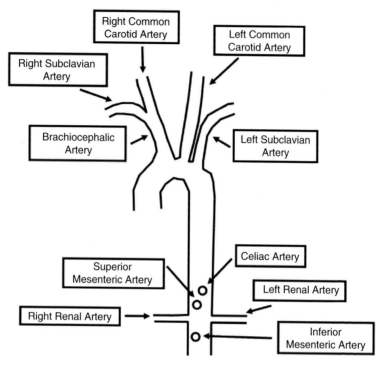

Figure 8.11. Normal anatomy of the aorta.

aortic arch where the ligamentum arteriosum has calcified), and coarctation. Soft plaque in the ascending aorta and aortic arch is associated with an increased stroke incidence (3 times as predictive as carotid artery disease) and, thus, soft plaque is more dangerous than calcified or hard plaque. Always look at the noncontrasted scan as well for calcium. Penetrating ulcers, intramural hematoma, and dissection may also be seen. Calcium in the lumen of an aorta with dissection indicates the true lumen. The false lumen is typically the bigger lumen. When evaluating aortic dissection, the initiation (entry point), ending point, involved arterial branches (i.e., subclavian artery, carotid artery, etc.), as well as the true versus false lumen must be identified. Vessels originating from the false lumen must be identified (i.e., coronary arteries, mesenteric arteries, renal arteries, etc.). The spectrum of disease in order of severity is as follows: penetrating ulcer, intramural hematoma, and dissection. Remember that thrombus density is approximately +50 Hounsfield units. Vasculitis such as Takayasu's arteritis may also be diagnosed (thick great vessel walls with dilation).

Pericardium

Be sure to assess the pericardium. There are three attachment points of the pericardium (base of the aorta, bottom frenulum of the diaphragm, small piece on the inside of the sternum). There is usually slack in the pericardium but in some patients the pericardium is taut and may be tacked to the sternum. This variant is associated with tethering and premature ventricular contractions. Describe the pericardium, commenting on the thickness (mild, moderate, or severe) and extent (focal, limited, or diffuse and extensive). The pericardium should be <4 mm thick. Also comment on the presence of pericardial calcification of the pericardium. The pericardium is often focally thick around the right atrium and this is a normal finding. Comment on the presence or absence of a pericardial effusion and its size and character. Pericardial fluid can be characterized by measuring the Hounsfield units. Thrombus and blood are +50. Transudate is <25 and exudate is >50. Look for the hemodynamic effects of the effusion (heart motion, impingement of chambers, etc.).

Pericardial Arteries and Veins

Pericardial arteries and veins may cause confusion when interpreting a cardiac CTA because they appear as contrasted vascular structures that run across the heart. If a contrasted vascular structure running over the heart with no apparent anatomic connection is seen, consider that this structure is a pericardial artery or vein.

Persistent Absence of the Left Pericardium

This condition is characterized by an absence of the pericardium over the left ventricle and results in adherence of the heart to the left-sided pleura. The myocardium can herniate through the hole.

Pulmonary Embolism

Pulmonary embolism is a significant cause of morbidity and mortality. Figure 8.12 illustrates a good example of a pulmonary embolism detected by CT. The PIOPED study[30] in 1990 indicated that 88% of patients with a high-probability V/Q scan had a pulmonary embolism but also 33% of patients with an intermediate V/Q scan and still 12% of patients with a low-risk V/Q scan had pulmonary embolis. Pulmonary angiography is invasive and carries an inherently increased risk. Multidetector CT is also a great technique to look

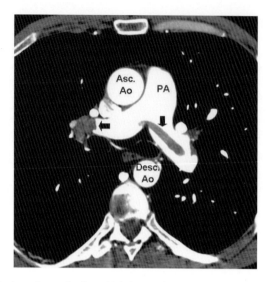

Figure 8.12. A good example of a multiple large pulmonary emboli (black arrows) depicted as filling defects void of contrast in the pulmonary artery (PA).

for pulmonary embolis. Antecubital vein contrast is injected at 3 cc/second. A preset delay of 15–20 seconds suffices in most patients. But, a test bolus may be used. Patients with negative pulmonary embolism CT studies and negative lower-extremity Doppler examinations for deep venous thrombosis, and in whom anticoagulation was held, have very low probability of pulmonary embolism over the next 3–6 months.[31]

When assessing a CT scan for pulmonary embolism, use thin slices and be sure to cover the lung apices in the sFOV. Follow the pulmonary arteries out as far as possible to rule out thrombus. Evaluate the size of the right heart and look for septal bowing. Recognize flow artifact in the veins and the right side of the heart. Using a triple injection technique described above may reduce flow artifact. Remember, the larger the scan field, the longer the breath hold (more artifacts), and the less contrast there will be at the bottom of the scan field. These limitations may decrease the ability to adequately visualize the coronary arteries. Everything in cardiac CT is a trade off.

The "triple rule out" is difficult but feasible. The technique would require a triphasic contrast bolus technique using an initial contrast bolus followed by a mix of contrast and saline followed by a saline chaser. This allows adequate visualization of the right heart and of the pulmonary arteries without compromising the left-sided evaluation of the coronary arteries and great vessels. There are negatives to the triple rule out technique. Radiation dose is much higher even with ECG pulsing because the sFOV is much greater, thereby increasing the scan time. In addition, the contrast dose is approximately 30%

higher. In the absence of clinical suspicion, it is rare to find occult pulmonary emboli or aortic dissections. Therefore, the "routine" triple rule out is not recommended.

Cardiac Masses

Cardiac masses including tumors, myxomas, thrombi, and vegetations (Figure 8.5) are easily seen using cardiac CTA. However, differentiating them may be challenging since their tissue density will be similar to the myocardium. For this reason, myxomas are often difficult to visualize in the noncontrasted scan since they tend to blend in with the normal heart tissue. However, myxomas will enhance after contrast is given and thus will appear brighter in the contrasted CTA. By manipulating the image plane, the attachment point of tumors and myxomas is easily identified.

Thrombi are also notable on CTA. First, an absence of contrast may be noted in the ventricular or atrial cavity in the location of the thrombus. Although a thrombus may have a density similar to normal tissue, its location and clinical setting (left atrial appendage in a large atrium in atrial fibrillation or in the ventricular apex in a patient with a thinned-out apex and previous myocardial infarction) will often be a clue to its presence.

Vegetations have tissue density similar to heart muscle as well. Again, their location, the clinical picture, and the size, shape, and smoothness of the vegetation borders may help to differentiate vegetations from normal tissue and other masses. Ring abscesses may also be visualized. Often, contrast dye will appear to be moving into a cavity where dye does not usually exist, in a location common to abscesses.

Liquefaction necrosis of mitral annular calcification is a noteworthy and potentially confusing finding. It will appear as a rounded density in the area of the mitral annulus with calcium and liquid density inside. Liquefaction necrosis may be large and if large enough, may compress the mitral valve and subsequently hinder mitral inflow. On echocardiogram, it appears as a rounded, echo-dense mass with smooth borders located in the periannular region with no acoustic shadowing artifacts. There are also central areas of echolucencies.

Right Ventricular Dysplasia

The key to diagnosing right ventricular dysplasia is to identify dilation and wall motion abnormalities of the right ventricle. Increased trabeculations and significant scalloping of the right ventricular free wall is a significant abnormal finding as well. In addition, fat density in the free wall of the right ventricle (-100 Hounsfield units) may also be identified. A mild amount of fat proximal to the moderator band is an acceptable variant. Fat present in more than 50% of the right ventricular free wall or fat seen distal to the moderator band are significantly abnormal findings. Magnetic resonance imaging remains the preferred imaging modality for this pathology but CTA is the second choice.

Cardiac Source of Embolism

Cardiac CTA is a reasonable test for cardiac source of embolism. The inferior vena cava may be seen all the way to the left atrium and shunts from the inferior vena cava to the left atrium that are not visible by TEE are potentially visualized by CTA. Sinus venosus atrial septal defects are easily identified as is anomalous pulmonary venous return. A patent foramen ovale is also easily seen. The left atrial appendage is beautifully visualized. Furthermore, the aorta, the carotid arteries, vertebral arteries, and possibly the intracranial vessels (if the sFOV is large enough) may be seen with the same imaging study. Finally, as noted above, cardiac masses such as myxomas are easily identified as possible embolic sources.[31]

Shunts

The flow of contrast through the aorta and pulmonary artery can be separately tracked and contrast density versus time curves may be generated for both the aorta and pulmonary artery. From these curves, shunt fractions can be calculated. Contrast timing delays may be identified in the case of a flow obstruction. In addition, a delayed secondary curve (second peak) may be seen if a shunt is present (Figure 8.13). In addition, analysis of the cardiac CTA images may identify dye flux moving between cardiac chambers.

Identifying a contrast jet moving from the left atrium into the right atrium easily identifies an atrial septal defect (Figure 8.14). Negative contrast in the

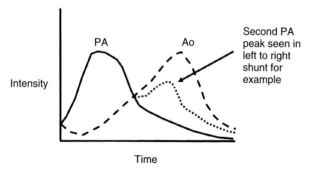

Figure 8.13. The use of flow intensity curves to evaluate intracardiac shunts by cardiac CTA. In this example, a left to right shunt is identified by the delayed secondary peak in the pulmonary artery (PA) contrast intensity curve. Ao, aorta.

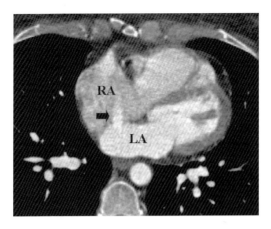

Figure 8.14. Flow (black arrow) from the left atrium (LA) to the right atrium (RA) indicative of a secundum atrial septal defect. Note that the RA is enlarged.

left atrium is also visualized if there is a right to left shunt. Figure 8.15 illustrates the location of various atrial septal defects. Closure devices are also seen. For example, the Amplatzer closure device has a typical CTA appearance (Figure 8.16). Cardiac CTA can also aid in defining the likelihood of successful placement of the Amplatzer closure device by defining the size of the atrial septal defect and the presence or absence of adequate tissue on either side of the defect, which is needed for device clamping and adherence. The classification and incidence of atrial septal defects are as follows. Ostium secundum occurs in 60%, ostium primum occurs in 20%, superior sinus venosus occurs in 15%, and inferior sinus venosus occurs in <5%. Coronary sinus atrial septal

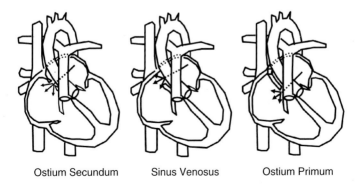

Ostium Secundum   Sinus Venosus   Ostium Primum

Figure 8.15. The location of various atrial septal defects.

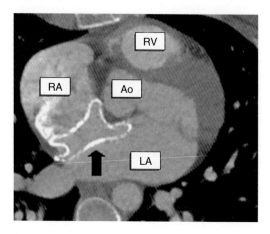

Figure 8.16. The typical cardiac CTA appearance of an Amplatzer atrial septal defect closure device (black arrow). RA, right atrium; RV, right ventricle; Ao, aorta; LA, left atrium.

defects occur in <1% and a true common atrium is seen in <5% of all atrial septal defects.

Ventricular septal defects of all types (membranous/perimembranous, muscular, inlet or outlet/supracristal) may also be well visualized. Figure 8.17 depicts the location of various ventricular septal defects.

Hypertrophic Obstructive Cardiomyopathy

Assess for asymmetric septal hypertrophy and for systolic anterior motion of the mitral valve.

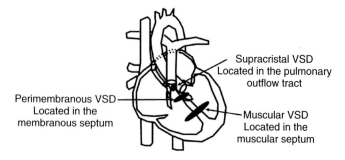

Figure 8.17. The location of various ventricular septal defects (VSDs).

Cardiac Compression Syndrome

Cardiac compression syndrome is a frequently unrecognized source of ill-described chest pain and palpitations. This condition is characterized by close proximity of the right ventricle to the sternum where the right heart is compressed against the sternum. Cardiac compression syndrome may be congenital or acquired. The anterior to posterior chest diameter may be congenitally narrow. In addition, the syndrome may be caused by an extra-cardiac mass pushing the heart anteriorly or by a hiatal hernia. In addition, cardiac chamber enlargement can produce this syndrome.

With the cardiac compression syndrome, the heart contacts the sternum and becomes irritated as it rubs against the anterior chest wall. The pericardium may become inflamed and a contact, focal pericarditis may ensue. In addition, the compressed heart may squeeze the valve planes together producing a variant of the so-called mitral valve prolapse syndrome. Tricuspid valve prolapse may also be seen. Because the right heart chambers are compressed, these patients may vagal easily because of compression of right ventricular filling.

The cardiac compression syndrome may manifest a large spectrum of symptoms including palpitations, atypical chest pain, light-headedness and fainting. In addition, because the heart is in contact with the chest wall, these patients may complain that they feel their heart beating. It should be noted that 2% of normal patients have their hearts in slight contact with the sternum while lying on their back. In chest pain patients, 10% have substantial areas of contact (Callister, The Tennessee Heart and Vascular Institute, unpublished oral communication, November 4, 2005).

Myocardial Noncompaction

During embryogenesis before the coronary arteries develop, the myocardium receives blood flow from endocardial sinusoids similar to a reptile. In some patients, these sinusoids remain in adulthood and appear as multiple trabeculations in the endocardial side of the left ventricular myocardium (not unlike the normal right ventricular appearance). These ventricles are prone to dilate and a dilated cardiomyopathy may ensue. This condition is well visualized with cardiac CTA.

Collateral Vessels

Collateral vessels are usually <1 mm in diameter and, thus, most often cannot be seen by cardiac CTA. Rarely, collaterals are visible but this is the exception and not the rule. Sometimes collateral vessels can be implied by distal visualization of an occluded vessel or visualization of a vessel with a subtotal occlusion. Subtotal stenoses cannot be differentiated from total occlusions with collateral flow. The more tortuous or winding an artery, the more likely it is a collateral vessel.

Coronary Anomalies

Coronary anomalies are present in up to 1.2% of the population and cause 12% of sports-related sudden deaths and 1.2% of non–sports-related sudden deaths.[32] Coronary anomalies have been implicated in chest pain, sudden death, cardiomyopathy, syncope, dyspnea, ventricular arrhythmias, and myocardial infarction.

Anomalies frequently causing ischemia include coronary fistulas, left main arising from the pulmonary artery, left main arising from the right coronary sinus, RCA arising from the left coronary sinus, and single coronary artery coursing between the aorta and pulmonary artery. Anomalies that do not cause ischemia include the circumflex arising from the right coronary sinus (always travels posterior to the aorta and therefore is a benign finding), absent left main (split origin of the LAD and circumflex), and high or low origin of the RCA. Figure 8.18 illustrates examples of common coronary anomalies.

When coronary artery anomalies are suspected and when assessing complex coronary anatomy, use thin MIP or MPR. Often the origin of the coronaries is among many overlapping structures and therefore thin MIP or MPR is best to define this anatomy.

If a coronary artery anomaly exists, a few anatomic questions must be answered. Is the anomalous coronary artery intramural or extramural (Figures 8.19 and 8.20)? Extramural is the usual course of a coronary artery. Intramural

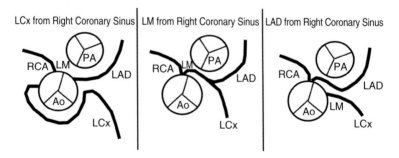

Figure 8.18. Three common coronary anomalies. The first anomaly is the left circumflex (LCx) artery originating from the right coronary cusp. The second anomaly is where the left main (LM) coronary artery arises from the right coronary cusp. The left main may course anterior to the pulmonary artery (PA), posterior to the aorta (Ao), or between the aorta and the pulmonary artery (the most malignant). The last anomaly is when the LAD coronary artery arises from the right coronary cusp and it may also travel anterior, posterior, or between the two great arteries. The normally arising left main in this case gives rise to the circumflex only.

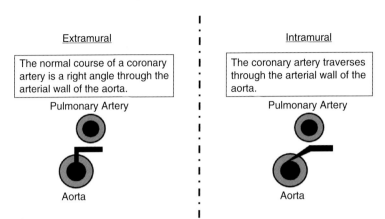

Extramural | Intramural

The normal course of a coronary artery is a right angle through the arterial wall of the aorta.

The coronary artery traverses through the arterial wall of the aorta.

Pulmonary Artery

Aorta

Pulmonary Artery

Aorta

Figure 8.19. An extramural versus intramural course of an anomalous coronary artery coursing between the pulmonary artery and the aorta. Usually, the coronary artery travels a perpendicular course through the aortic wall as it leaves the aorta. An intramural coursing anomalous artery travels diagonally through the aortic wall as it exits, resulting in a pinpoint origin of the artery, which is a negative prognosticator for cardiac events such as angina and sudden cardiac death.

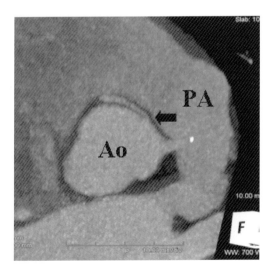

Figure 8.20. A good example of an intramural anomalous right coronary artery. Note the "slit-like" origin, the acute angle take off, and the asymmetric course as the artery traverses between the aorta (Ao) and pulmonary artery (PA).

anomalous coronary arteries place patients at higher risk for symptoms such as dyspnea, angina, and sudden death. Three criteria must be fulfilled to diagnose an intramural course to a coronary anomaly. First, a slit-like, narrow ostium must be noted. Second, an acute angle take off of the coronary artery from the aorta must be identified (the usual origin of a coronary artery is that of a right angle take off), and lastly, the coronary artery must be asymmetrically positioned between the aorta and the pulmonary artery. That is, the space from the aorta to the position of the coronary is less than the space between the coronary and the pulmonary artery. All three criteria must be present to definitively diagnose an intramural course to an anomalous coronary artery (Shen, et al. Cleveland Clinic, Ft. Lauderdale, unpublished written communication, January 26, 2006). Because of the acute take-off angle and slit-like origin of the anomaly, a special catheter called a LIYA is often needed to engage an intramural anomalous coronary artery during invasive angiography.

The treatment of choice for an intramural coronary anomaly is unroofing surgery (Figure 8.21). A hole is placed through the wall of the aorta to directly connect the lumen of the aortic to the coronary artery lumen. A wire probe is placed in the intramural anomalous coronary artery and the surgeon palpates the common wall between the coronary and the aorta. A hole is then made to connect the two arteries. The hole is sutured around its periphery to prevent clotting off of the connection. In emergency cases, stenting can be done because the wall of the aorta is elastic and, thus, if not calcified it is unlikely to dissect during stent placement.

The second question that must be answered when a coronary anomaly is identified is the course of the artery. Is the coronary artery running between the pulmonary artery and the aorta, behind the aorta, or in front of the pulmonary artery? Figure 7.5 (see page 85) demonstrates an anomalous left main coronary artery traversing between the pulmonary artery and aorta. Anomalies that course between the great vessels pose higher risk for serious symptoms, possibly because of compression or irritation of the artery as the great vessels engorge during exercise or because of a very narrow (slit-like) ostium.

Next, determine whether the artery is intramuscular versus extramuscular. An intramuscular course, particularly when the artery runs within the interventricular septum, is less malignant.

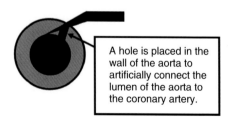

A hole is placed in the wall of the aorta to artificially connect the lumen of the aorta to the coronary artery.

Figure 8.21. The unroofing procedure for correcting an intramural coursing anomalous coronary artery.

Several clinical questions should also be considered. The answers are determined by a thorough history, physical examination, and by further clinical testing. The answers to these questions determine further treatment. Is their ischemia? Is there arrhythmia? That is, does the patient have chest pain, syncope, or palpitations? A Holter monitor may be placed, a stress test at 100% maximum predicted heart rate with no β-blockers may be performed (looking for exercise-induced angina or arrhythmia such as ventricular tachycardia or premature ventricular contractions) and finally, if necessary, an electrophysiology study may help. Rarely, a dobutamine echocardiogram may be performed in the catheterization laboratory to look for compression of the arteries during physiologic stress. These abnormalities represent a spectrum of symptoms and the treatments vary from β-blockade to defibrillators to corrective surgery.

Myocardial Bridges

Myocardial bridges are common (seen in approximately 5% of all CTA examinations). They occur exclusively in the LAD artery. In this condition, a segment of the coronary artery runs intramuscularly. The artery is called a tunneled artery. During systole, there is compression of the artery. Because most coronary filling occurs during diastole, the majority of clinical cases are asymptomatic and usually coronary flow is not diminished. Rarely there is association with myocardial ischemia, perfusion abnormalities, and chest pain. Bridges are best seen in short-axis views where the artery is in cross-section. The LAD artery is seen diving into the myocardium as the reader scrolls through the slices. Often, the major septal perforator will be absent since it is replaced by the intramyocardial LAD arterial segment. The diagnosis should not be made unless confirmed in the short-axis view.

Thoracic Aortic Anomalies

These anomalies are explained by persistence of a segment of the aortic arch that should have regressed or regression of a segment that should have persisted. Although rare, those that participate in cardiac CTA should be aware of these abnormalities.

Left Arch with Aberrant Right Subclavian Artery

This anomaly is the most common congenital abnormality of the aortic arch vessels (Figure 8.22). The right subclavian artery is the last of the major arteries to arise from the aortic arch. The order of the great vessels in this

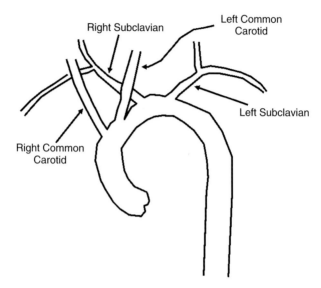

Figure 8.22. An aberrant right subclavian artery originating from a normal left-sided aortic arch.

anomaly moving distally along the aorta is right common carotid, left common carotid, left subclavian, and then right subclavian, which courses obliquely behind the trachea and esophagus to reach the right arm. This is usually an asymptomatic anomaly. However, a tortuous aberrant right subclavian artery may compress the esophagus and cause dysphagia. There may also be a right rather than left ligamentum arteriosum causing a vascular ring around the esophagus or trachea, resulting in shortness of breath or dysphagia.

Right Aortic Arch Anomalies

The two types of right aortic arch anomalies include a right aortic arch with aberrant left subclavian artery (more common in adults), and a right aortic arch with mirror-image branching (more common in children). In the right arch with aberrant left subclavian artery, the great arteries originate from the arch in the following order: left common carotid, right common carotid, right subclavian artery, and left subclavian artery. The descending aorta is more often right sided. If the ligamentum arteriosum is on the left, a vascular ring can form and there may be resulting symptoms.

In the right arch with mirror imaging, the great arteries originate in the following order: left innominate artery, right carotid, and right subclavian. The descending aorta is usually on the right. These patients are usually children and have associated cyanotic heart disease, including tetralogy of Fallot, truncus arteriosus, pulmonary artery atresia with ventricular septal defect, tricuspid atresia, double outlet right ventricle, and transposition of the great arteries.

Double Aortic Arch

This anomaly is characterized by two aortic arches arising from a single ascending aorta. Each arch gives rise to its own subclavian and carotid artery before becoming a single descending aorta, which is usually left sided. The right arch is typically larger and more cephalad than the left arch. These patients often have esophageal or tracheal compression.

Cervical Aortic Arch

This is a rare anomaly characterized by a high-riding, elongated aortic arch extending cephalad in the mediastinum before turning downward. The arch often projects above the level of the clavicles. Associated findings are often absence of the innominate artery, origin of the contralateral subclavian artery from the descending proximal aorta, and a retroesophageal course of the descending aorta with the descending aorta lying on the right side contralateral to the arch. If the ligamentum arteriosum is on the opposite side of the arch, a vascular ring will form and cause symptoms. If not, the patient is asymptomatic.

Coarctation

Coarctation of the aorta is found in 5%–8% of the population.[33] Two major types include preductal (infantile) and postductal (adult). The preductal form occurs immediately below the origin of the left subclavian artery at the insertion of the ductus arteriosus or ligamentum arteriosum. This type is usually associated with a long segment narrowing or hypoplasia of the transverse aortic arch and with congenital heart lesions including ventricular septal defect, patent ductus arteriosus, and hypoplastic left heart. A preductal coarctation of the aorta usually presents within 6 months of birth with congestive heart failure.

The postductal form is more common and is located at the junction of the distal aortic arch and the descending aorta, immediately below the obliterated ductus arteriosus. The coarctation is usually localized. The ascending aorta is usually dilated and postcoarctation dilation of the descending aorta is usually noted. Large intercostal and internal thoracic arteries establish collateral circulation between the proximal and distal parts of the aorta. Therefore, rib notching may be seen. Postductal coarctation of the aorta is usually found by evaluating patients for hypertension or when evaluating patients with a bicuspid aortic valve, which is found in 1%–2% of the population.[34] Coarctation of the aorta is identified in up to 85% of patients with a bicuspid aortic valve.[35] Blood pressure is usually higher in the upper extremities than the lower extremities. If there is a concomitant aberrant right subclavian artery, the pressure in the right upper extremity may be lower than the left.

Identification of collaterals is crucial because if there are insufficient collaterals, cross-clamping of the aorta may result in spinal cord ischemia. The presence of more extensive collaterals suggests that the coarctation is clinically significant. Recurrent coarctation of the aorta after repair occurs in 5%–30% of repair patients.[33]

Interruption of the Aortic Arch

This anomaly is very rare. It is related to regression of portions of the aortic arch on two sides. Type A is interruption distal to the left subclavian. Type B is interruption between the left common carotid and left subclavian. Type C is interruption between the brachiocephalic trunk and the left carotid. A dilated ductus arteriosus supplies the descending aorta beyond the interruption and may be mistaken for the aortic arch itself. Most aortic arch interruptions present early in life with respiratory distress, cyanosis, and congestive heart failure. Congenital heart disease is usually present and includes ventricular septal defect, bicuspid aortic valve, aortopulmonary window, double-outlet right ventricle, and single ventricle.

Aortopulmonary Anomalies

Truncus Arteriosus

Truncus arteriosus results from failure of proximal division of the aorta and pulmonary artery. Therefore, in these patients, the pulmonary and systemic systems arise from a common trunk. Type I is a common trunk with confluent pulmonary arteries. Type II is a common trunk with absence of one pulmonary artery. Type III is a common trunk with interrupted aortic arch or severe coarctation.

Hemitruncus Arteriosus

In this anomaly, one of the pulmonary arteries originates from the ascending aorta. The other arises from the right ventricle. These patients present in infancy with congestive heart failure.

Patent Ductus Arteriosus

The ductus arteriosus represents persistence of the distal part of the aortic arch. In most patients, the ductus closes shortly after birth by contraction of the muscular wall. A patent ductus arteriosus will appear on CTA as a small tubular structure connecting the descending aorta with the distal main pulmonary artery or with the proximal left pulmonary artery. Treatment is device closure or operative repair.

Aortopulmonary Window

An aortopulmonary window is a direct communication between the proximal ascending aorta and the main pulmonary artery. This rare anomaly results from incomplete division of the common arterial trunk. Most patients are diagnosed in infancy when they present with congestive heart failure. If the lesion is small, it may not be diagnosed until later in life. Treatment is surgical with suturing or a patch.

Transposition of the Great Arteries

Complete transposition (D-transposition) is characterized by discordant connection of the great arteries and the ventricles such that the pulmonary artery arises from the left ventricle and the aorta arises from the right ventricle and there is usually an associated ventricular septal defect. This lesion causes cyanosis at birth. Corrected transposition (L-transposition) is characterized by double discordance, both ventriculoarterial and atrioventricular, resulting in normal physiologic flow of blood. Here, the pulmonary artery arises from the anatomic left ventricle and the aorta arises from the anatomic right ventricle. In addition, the left atrium connects the right ventricle and the right atrium connects to the left ventricle. Thus, blood from the right atrium goes through a right-sided left ventricle to the lungs. Blood from the left atrium goes through a left-sided right ventricle to the aorta and out to the systemic circulation. These patients have arrhythmogenic problems and later in life develop failure of the anatomic right ventricle.

On CTA, the aorta usually lies anterior and to the right of the pulmonary artery. The Mustard procedure is used to correct this problem and uses a baffle to direct the venous blood flow to the venous atrium (blood from the venous side to the left atrium). On CTA, if the superior vena cava is followed downward, the baffle will be seen crossing the atrial septum and diverting blood into the left atrium. It is common to see pacemakers in these patients because they frequently experience bradyarrhythmias. If the coronary arteries arise from the pulmonary artery, they will need to be reimplanted.

Pulmonary Artery Anomalies

Idiopathic Dilation of the Pulmonary Artery Trunk

Idiopathic dilation of the pulmonary artery trunk refers to enlargement of the pulmonary outflow track without pulmonary valvular stenosis. This finding is usually incidental.

Absence or Proximal Interruption of the Pulmonary Artery

In these anomalies, interruption of the right or left pulmonary artery is usually seen within 1 cm of its origin from the main pulmonary artery. The distal vessels are frequently diminutive and supplied by systemic collaterals. Pulmonary venous drainage is normal. The associated lung is usually small. There are many other congenital anomalies that usually coexist with this finding and therefore absence or proximal interruption of the pulmonary artery is often diagnosed early in life.

Pulmonary Artery Stenosis

Pulmonary artery stenosis can occur anywhere from the pulmonary valve to the peripheral arteries. It can be single or multiple and unilateral or bilateral. Central and peripheral stenoses can occur in combination. This anomaly is often associated with Williams syndrome, Noonan's syndrome, and Ehlers-Danlos syndrome.

Pulmonary Sling

In the case of a pulmonary sling, the left pulmonary artery originates from the right pulmonary artery and crosses the mediastinum, extending between the trachea and esophagus to reach the left hilum. The anomolous artery can cause a compressive effect on the airway.

Pulmonary Venous Anomalies

Total Anomalous Pulmonary Venous Return

Here, the pulmonary veins connect to a systemic venous structure, which returns the blood to the right heart. An atrial septal defect allows mixing of oxygenated and deoxygenated blood. Total anomalous pulmonary venous return can be supracardiac, cardiac, infracardiac, or mixed. Pulmonary venous obstruction is usually present in the infracardiac form. Patients present early in life with cyanosis.

Partial Anomalous Venous Connection

This anomaly produces a left to right shunt. Right-sided partial anomalous pulmonary venous return is twice as common as left sided. Three patterns are noted: anomalous right superior pulmonary venous drainage to the superior vena cava, anomalous left superior pulmonary venous return into a left brachiocephalic vein or innominate vein, and anomalous right lower lobe drainage into the inferior vena cava or portal vein.

Pulmonary Varix

A varicosity of a pulmonary vein may be congenital or present as result of chronic pulmonary hypertension. Patients may be asymptomatic or present with hemoptysis.

Systemic Thoracic Venous Anomalies

Persistent Left Superior Vena Cava

A persistent left superior vena cava lies anterior to the left subclavian artery and lateral to the left common carotid. It passes lateral to the aortic arch as it descends. It also courses lateral to the main pulmonary artery and anterior to the hilum. Most frequently, it drains into the coronary sinus. A clue to its existence is an enlarged coronary sinus.

Azygous Continuation of the Inferior Vena Cava

This anomaly results when the suprarenal segment of the inferior vena cava fails to develop. Thus, blood from the lower half of the body is returned to the heart via the retrocrural azygous and hemiazygous veins, which are derived from the right supracardinal vein. Often this is an incidental, asymptomatic finding. CTA findings will show a dilated azygous arch and a dilated azygous vein.

Coronary Artery Fistulas and Other Cardiac Fistulas

CTA is very good at identifying fistulas. The most common fistulas empty into right-sided structures such as the coronary sinus and right atrium. The important strength of cardiac CTA is the ability to manipulate the image planes and move through image slices to identify the origin, the course, and the end point of these vascular structures.

References

1. Arad Y, Goodman K, Roth M, et al. Coronary calcification, coronary disease risk factors, C-reactive protein, and atherosclerotic cardiovascular disease events. The St. Francis Heart Study. J Am Coll Cardiol 2005;46(1):158–165.
2. Taylor AJ, Bindeman J, Feuerstein I, et al. Coronary artery calcium independently predicts incident premature coronary heart disease over measured cardiovascular risk factors: mean three-year outcomes in the Prospective Army Coronary Calcium (PACC) Project. J Am Coll Cardiol 2005;46(5):807–814.
3. Berman DS, Wong ND, Gransar H, et al. Relationship between stress-induced myocardial ischemia and atherosclerosis measured by coronary calcium tomography. J Am Coll Cardiol 2004;44(4):923–930.
4. Shaw LJ, Raggi P, Schisterman E, Berman DS, Callister TQ. Prognostic value of cardiac risk factors and coronary artery calcium screening for all cause mortality. Radiology 2003;228:826–833.
5. Lamant DH, Budoff MJ, Shavelle DM, et al. Coronary calcium scanning adds incremental value to patients with positive stress tests. Am Heart J 2002;143(5): 861–867.
6. Haberl R, Tittus J, Czernik A, et al. Multislice spiral computed tomographic angiography of coronary arteries in patients with suspected coronary artery disease: an effective filter before catheter angiography? Am Heart J 2005;149(6):960–961.
7. Rumberger JA, Sheedy PF, Breen JF, Schwartz RS. Coronary calcium, as determined by electron beam computed tomography, and coronary disease on arteriogram. Effect of patient's sex on diagnosis. Circulation 1995;91(5):1363–1367.
8. Knez A, Becker A, Leber A, et al. Relation of coronary calcium scores by electron beam tomography to obstructive disease in 2115 symptomatic patients. Am J Cardiol 2004;93(9):1150–1152.
9. Lauden DA, Vukov LF, Breen JF, et al. Use of electron beam computed tomography in the evaluation of chest pain patients in the emergency department. Ann Emerg Med 1999;33(1):15–21.
10. Wayhs R, Zelinger A, Raggi P. High coronary artery calcium scores pose an extremely elevated risk for hard events. J Am Coll Cardiol 2002;39(2):225–230.
11. Budoff MJ, Shavelle DM, Lamont D, et al. Usefulness of electron beam computed tomography scanning for distinguishing ischemic from nonischemic cardiomyopathy. J Am Coll Cardiol 1998;34(5):1173–1178.
12. Budoff MJ, Jacob B, Rasouli ML, Yu D, et al. Comparison of electron beam computed tomography and technetium stress testing in differentiating cause of dilated versus ischemic cardiomyopathy. J Comput Assist Tomogr 2005;29(5):699–703.
13. Le T, Ko JY, Kim HT, et al. Comparison of echocardiography and electron beam tomography in differentiating the etiology of heart failure. Clin Cardiol 2000;23(6): 417–420.

14. Raggi P, Callister TQ, Shaw LJ. Progression of coronary artery calcium and risk of first myocardial infarction in patients receiving cholesterol-lowering therapy. Arterioscler Thromb Vasc Biol 2004;24(7):1272–1277.

15. Kalia NK, Miller LG, Nasir K, et al. Visualizing coronary calcium is associated with improvements in adherence to statin therapy. Atherosclerosis 2006;185(2):394–399.

16. Takasu J, Shavelle DM, O'Brien KD, et al. Association between progression of aortic valve calcification and coronary calcification: assessment by electron beam tomography. Acad Radiol 2005;12(3):298–304.

17. CCT/CMR Writing Group. ACCF/ACR/SCCT/SCMR/ASNC/NASCI/SCAI/SIR appropriateness criteria for cardiac computed tomography and cardiac magnetic resonance. J Am Coll Cardiol 2006;48(7):1–21.

17A. Ambrose JA, Fuster V. The risk of coronary occlusion is not proportional to the prior severity of coronary stenosis. Heart 1998;79(1):3–4.

18. Garcia MJ, Lessick J, Hoffman MH, et al. Accuracy of 16-row multidetector computed tomography for the assessment of coronary artery stenosis. JAMA 2006;296(4):403–411.

19. Flohr TG, McCollough CH, Bruder H, et al. First performance evaluation of a dual-source CT (DSCT) system. Eur Radiol 2006;16(2):256–268.

20. Gaspar T, Halon D, Rubinshtein R, Peled N. Clinical applications and future trends in cardiac CTA. Eur Radiol 2005;15(suppl 4):D10–14.

21. Yonetsu T, Kakuta T, Kimura S, et al. Coronary artery lesions with intra-plaque enhancement in multidetector spiral computed tomography [abstract]. J Am Coll Cardiol. February 21, 2006;47(4) Suppl A: Abstract 970–976.

22. Meyer TS, Hausleiter J, Huber E, et al. Influence of scan protocols on radiation dose estimates for coronary 64-slice computed tomography angiography [abstract]. J Am Coll Cardiol. February 21, 2006;47(4) Suppl A: Abstract 807–813.

22A. Thompson RC, Cullom SJ. Issues regarding radiation dosage of cardiac nuclear and radiography procedures. J Nucl Cardiol 2006;13(1):19–23.

23. Einstein AJ, Sanz J, Dellegrottaglie S, et al. Radiation dose and predictable cancer risk in multidetector-row computed tomography angiography [abstract]. J Am Coll Cardiol. February 21, 2006;47(4) Suppl A: Abstract 807–817.

24. Achenbach S, Ropers D, Holle J, et al. In-plane coronary arterial motion velocity: measurement with electron-beam CT. Radiology 2000;216(2):457–463.

25. Baks T, Cademartiri F, Moelker AD, et al. Multislice computed tomography and magnetic resonance imaging for the assessment of reperfused acute myocardial infarction. J Am Coll Cardiol 2006;48(1):144–152.

26. George RT, Silva C, Cordeiro MA, et al. Multidetector computed tomography myocardial perfusion imaging during adenosine stress. J Am Coll Cardiol 2006;48(1):153–160.

27. MacMahon H, Austin JH, Gamsu G, et al. Guidelines for management of small pulmonary nodules detected on CT scans: a statement from the Fleischner society. Radiology 2005;237(2):395–400.

28. Caragher TE, Fernandez BB, Barr LA. Long-term experience with an accelerated protocol for diagnosis of chest pain. Arch Pathol Lab Med 2000;124(10):1434–1439.

29. Fynn SP, Kalman JM. Pulmonary veins: anatomy, electrophysiology, tachycardia, and fibrillation. Pacing Clin Electrophysiol 2004;27(11):1547–1559.

30. PIOPED Investigators. Value of the ventilation/perfusion scan in acute pulmonary embolism. Results of the prospective investigation of pulmonary embolism diagnosis (PIOPED). JAMA 1990;263(20):2753–2759.

31. Kavanagh EC, O'Hare A, Hargaden G, Murray JG. Risk of pulmonary embolism after negative MDCT pulmonary angiography findings. AJR Am J Roentgenol 2004;182(2):499–504.

32. von Kodolitsch Y, Franzen O, Lund GK, et al. Coronary artery anomalies. Part II. Recent insights from clinical investigations. Z Kardiol 2005;94(1):1–13.

33. Rao PS. Coarctation of the aorta. Curr Cardiol Rep 2005;7(6):425–434.

34. Braverman AC, Guven H, Beardslee MA, et al. The bicuspid aortic valve. Curr Probl Cardiol 2005;30(9):470–522.

35. Cury RC, Ferencik M, Achenbach S, et al. Accuracy of 16-slice multi-detector CT to quantify the degree of coronary artery stenosis: assessment of cross-sectional and longitudinal vessel reconstructions. Eur J Radiol 2006;57(3):345–350.

36. Achenbach S, Ropers D, Pohle FK, et al. Detection of coronary artery stenosis using multi-detector CT with 16 × 0.75 collimation and 375 ms rotation. Eur Heart J 2005;26(19):1978–1986.

37. Kuettner A, Beck T, Drosch T, et al. Image quality and diagnostic accuracy of noninvasive coronary imaging with 16 detector slice spiral computed tomography with 188 ms temporal resolution. Heart 2005;91(7):938–941.

38. Mollet NR, Cademartiri F, de Feyter PJ. Non-invasive multi-slice CT coronary imaging. Heart 2005;91:401–407.

39. Leber AW, Becker A, Kenz A, et al. Accuracy of 64-slice computed tomography to classify and quantify plaque volumes in the proximal coronary system: a comparative study using intravascular ultrasound. J Am Cardiol 2006;47(3):672–677.

40. Leschka S, Alkadhi H, Plass A, et al. Accuracy of MSCT coronary angiography with 64-slice technology: first experience. Eur Heart J 2005;26(15):1482–1787.

41. Raff G, Gallagher MJ, O'Neill WW, et al. Diagnostic accuracy of noninvasive coronary angiography using 64-slice spiral computed tomography. J Am Coll Cardiol 2005;46(3):522–557.

42. Pugliese F, Mollet NR, Runza G, et al. Diagnostic accuracy of non-invasive 64-slice CT coronary angiography in patients with stable angina pectoris. Eur Radiol 2006;16(3):575–582.

Index

Author Biographies

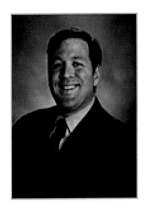

Dr. Pelberg graduated from Northwestern Medical School and completed a cardiology fellowship at the University of Virginia. He is level III certified in Cardiac CTA as recognized by The Society of Cardiovascular Computed Tomography. Currently, Dr. Pelberg practices cardiology at The Ohio Heart and Vascular Center.

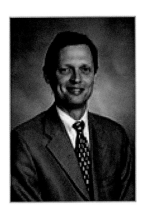

Dr. Mazur received his medical education at the Medical Academy in Poznan, Poland. He completed his cardiology fellowship at Baylor College of Medicine in Houston, Texas. Dr. Mazur is level III certified in Cardiac CTA as recognized by The Society of Cardiovascular Computed Tomography. Currently, Dr. Mazur practices cardiology at the Ohio Heart and Vascular Center.

Printed in Singapore